Personalized Medicine for Otolaryngology (ENT)

Personalized Medicine for Otolaryngology (ENT)

Guest Editor

Mehdi Abouzari

MDPI

Basel • Beijing • Wuhan • Barcelona • Belgrade • Novi Sad • Cluj • Manchester

Guest Editor
Mehdi Abouzari
Department of
Otolaryngology-Head and
Neck Surgery
University of California
Irvine
USA

Editorial Office
MDPI AG
Grosspeteranlage 5
4052 Basel, Switzerland

This is a reprint of the Special Issue, published open access by the journal *Journal of Personalized Medicine* (ISSN 2075-4426), freely accessible at: https://www.mdpi.com/journal/jpm/special_issues/MVQ66BX39O.

For citation purposes, cite each article independently as indicated on the article page online and as indicated below:

Lastname, A.A.; Lastname, B.B. Article Title. *Journal Name* **Year**, *Volume Number*, Page Range.

ISBN 978-3-7258-8033-1 (Hbk)
ISBN 978-3-7258-8034-8 (PDF)
https://doi.org/10.3390/books978-3-7258-8034-8

Contents

About the Editor

Mehdi Abouzari

Mehdi Abouzari, MD, PhD, is a translational physician–scientist, an assistant professor of otolaryngology, and director of clinical research of otology and neurotology at the University of California, Irvine. In addition to his clinical and research roles, Dr. Abouzari serves as an Associate Fellow of the American Neurotology Society, Associate Editor of *Frontiers in Audiology* and Otology, and Editorial Board Member of *Research in Vestibular Science*. He has authored over 125 peer-reviewed papers, 13 book chapters, and 2 books, and presented 120 abstracts at national and international conferences, with his work having received over 2500 citations to date. His most impactful work has been a group of studies showing that a number of ear disorders represent migraine phenomena. He has successfully led several clinical trials on the development of technology-based platforms and devices that address hearing loss and tinnitus. As director of the ENTelligence Lab, Dr. Abouzari pioneers the application of artificial intelligence and machine learning in otolaryngology and hearing sciences. His innovative approach combines traditional clinical expertise with advanced computational methods to develop new diagnostic and therapeutic solutions for patients with ear, nose, and throat conditions. Through this work, he is helping to shape the future of precision medicine in otolaryngology.

Journal of
Personalized Medicine

MDPI

orial

ɹrsonalized Medicine in Otolaryngology: Reflections on a ultidisciplinary Special Issue

hdi Abouzari

Division of Neurotology and Skull Base Surgery, Department of Otolaryngology-Head and Neck Surgery, University of California, Irvine, CA 92697, USA; mabouzar@hs.uci.edu; Tel.: +1-714-509-6096

1. Introduction

The practice of medicine has long aspired to treat the individual rather than the disease, yet it has only been in recent decades that the scientific and technological tools required to fulfill this aspiration have begun to mature [1]. In otolaryngology—a specialty that encompasses the remarkably diverse domains of oncology, neurotology, rhinology, laryngology, audiology, and head and neck surgery—the translation of personalized medicine principles into daily clinical practice carries particular relevance. The anatomical complexity, functional intimacy, and profound quality-of-life implications associated with disorders of the ear, nose, throat, and related structures make the "one-size-fits-all" paradigm especially inadequate. It was with this conviction that the present Special Issue was conceived: to gather original research, systematic reviews, consensus statements, and clinical trials that collectively advance our understanding of how individualized approaches can transform outcomes across all subspecialties of otolaryngology.

This closing editorial reflects on the eleven contributions that have shaped this Special Issue, acknowledging the breadth of the methodology, clinical scope, and translational ambition that they represent, and looking ahead to the horizon that their findings illuminate.

2. Head and Neck Oncology: From Population Trends to Precision Surgery

Two contributions in this Special Issue directly address the oncological domain, each from a distinct but complementary vantage point. The study by Lin and Hung on the diagnostic gap between clinical and pathological extranodal extension (ENE) in head and neck cancers represents a timely and methodologically rigorous contribution (Contribution 1). Using a five-year nationwide trend analysis from Taiwan, the authors expose a persistent and clinically consequential discordance between radiological or clinical staging and histopathological findings. Given that ENE is among the most powerful prognostic determinants in head and neck squamous cell carcinoma—driving decisions regarding adjuvant chemoradiation, surgical margins, and overall treatment intensity—this gap carries direct implications for individualized treatment planning [2]. The population-level scope of the analysis lends robustness to these findings and underscores the need for improved imaging protocols, intraoperative assessment tools, and perhaps molecular biomarkers that are capable of bridging this diagnostic divide.

Advancing personalized oncological care from a surgical perspective, the work on transoral cordectomy with microelectrodes (TOMES) on an outpatient basis demonstrates the feasibility of leveraging predictive models to tailor the perioperative experience for patients with early-stage laryngeal disease (Contribution 2). By integrating outcome prediction into the decision-making process for outpatient versus inpatient surgical pathways, this study exemplifies how data-driven personalization can simultaneously enhance patient comfort, streamline resource utilization, and maintain oncological safety. The incorporation of microelectrode technology into cordectomy further reflects the broader trajectory of precision surgical instrumentation in the specialty.

3. Neurotology and Inner Ear Disorders: Tailoring Rehabilitation and Therapy

The neurotological contributions to this Special Issue are notable both for their clinical relevance and for the heterogeneity of approaches that they employ. The manuscript on personalized vestibular assessment in older patients with cochlear implants addresses one of the more nuanced challenges at the intersection of auditory rehabilitation and balance medicine (Contribution 3). Cochlear implantation is well-established as a transformative intervention for severe-to-profound sensorineural hearing loss, yet its effects on vestibular function—particularly in an aging population that is already predisposed to multifactorial disequilibrium—deserve careful individual characterization [3]. The authors' call for tailored vestibular assessment protocols in this cohort not only refines candidacy evaluation and preoperative counseling but also informs postoperative rehabilitation strategies, underscoring that successful implantation extends beyond audiological outcomes alone.

Equally innovative is the proposal to repurpose SGLT-2 inhibitors as a novel therapeutic strategy for treatment-resistant Menière's disease (Contribution 4). Menière's disease remains one of the most therapeutically challenging conditions in otolaryngology, with a subset of patients failing conventional diuretic, dietary, and intratympanic interventions. By drawing on the well-characterized endolymphatic-decompressing and anti-inflammatory properties of sodium–glucose cotransporter-2 inhibitors—a drug class that was originally developed for glycemic control in type 2 diabetes—this contribution represents a paradigmatic example of pharmacological repurposing guided by pathophysiological reasoning. In an era where personalized pharmacotherapy increasingly incorporates comorbidity profiling and metabolic phenotyping, this proposal invites prospective investigation and may open a novel therapeutic corridor for a historically underserved patient population.

4. Rhinology and Sinonasal Disease: Evidence Synthesis and Consensus Building

The rhinological contributions to this Special Issue are united by a commitment to evidence synthesis and the formalization of clinical decision-making in complex scenarios. The systematic review of endoscopic sinus surgery in a frontal sinus inverted papilloma provides a comprehensive appraisal of surgical approaches, recurrence rates, and oncological outcomes in a condition characterized by significant anatomical variability and malignant transformation risk (Contribution 5). The findings reinforce the importance of individualized surgical planning—accounting for tumor origin, Krouse staging, frontal sinus anatomy, and surgeon experience—as determinants of both radicality and functional preservation.

The Young-IfOS consensus on the comprehensive management of cocaine-induced midline destructive lesions (CIMDL) addresses a clinically under-recognized yet growing entity that demands a highly personalized, multidisciplinary approach (Contribution 6). The destructive potential of CIMDL, combined with the psychiatric, social, and immunological complexity of affected patients, renders standardized treatment algorithms insufficient [4]. The consensus framework developed by an international panel of young otolaryngologists provides a valuable decision-support tool while explicitly accommodating patient-specific variables including addiction status, the extent of tissue destruction, immune profile, and psychosocial circumstances. The involvement of a junior faculty consortium also signals a generational commitment to advancing personalized care paradigms in rhinology.

https://doi.org/10.3390/jpm1605(

5. Audiology and Hearing Rehabilitation: Digital Health and Cognitive Horizons

Two contributions in this Special Issue explore the intersection of audiology with digital health and cognitive medicine, respectively, each reflecting the expanding scope of personalized audiological care. The systematic review and meta-analysis of internet-based therapies for tinnitus synthesizes evidence from randomized controlled trials to evaluate the efficacy of digital cognitive behavioral therapy (CBT), mindfulness-based interventions, and other web-delivered programs in this highly prevalent and quality-of-life-impairing condition (Contribution 7). Tinnitus affects a significant proportion of the adult population, yet access to specialized audiological and psychological care remains inequitable. Internet-delivered therapies hold particular promise in democratizing access to evidence-based intervention, and the granular analysis of effect sizes across outcome domains—tinnitus distress, anxiety, depression, and sleep quality—provides a nuanced basis for matching digital therapeutic modalities to individual patient profiles [5,6].

The study examining the association between hearing aid use and cognitive function in persons with hearing impairment, stratified by cardiovascular risk, addresses one of the most consequential questions in contemporary audiology (Contribution 8). The growing body of evidence linking untreated hearing loss to accelerated cognitive decline has elevated hearing rehabilitation from a quality-of-life intervention to a potential neuroprotective strategy. By stratifying outcomes according to cardiovascular risk—a well-established cognitive comorbidity—the authors contribute important nuance to the personalization of hearing aid prescription and counseling. The findings suggest that the cognitive benefits of amplification may be modulated by vascular health status: a finding with meaningful implications for the integrated management of older patients.

6. Laryngology and Voice Medicine: Electrophysiological Phenotyping

The characterization of the normal male and female voice using surface electromyographic (sEMG) parameters represents a foundational contribution to the laryngological component of this Special Issue (Contribution 9). Voice disorders are among the most functionally disabling conditions managed within otolaryngology, affecting professional voice users, patients recovering from laryngeal surgery, and individuals with neurological disease, among others. The establishment of normative sEMG profiles stratified by biological sex provides a critical reference framework for the objective, electrophysiological characterization of dysphonia—complementing acoustic and aerodynamic analyses and paving the way for individualized voice rehabilitation protocols. As artificial intelligence and machine learning tools increasingly enter the diagnostic landscape of laryngology, normative datasets such as those presented here become foundational infrastructure for personalized voice medicine.

7. Perioperative Care: Individualized Analgesia After Oropharyngeal Surgery

The randomized, double-blind trial evaluating pain after licorice or sugar–water gargling in patients recovering from oropharyngeal surgery contributes to the underexplored but clinically important domain of personalized perioperative analgesia (Contribution 10). Postoperative pain following tonsillectomy, uvulopalatopharyngoplasty, and related procedures remains a primary determinant of patient satisfaction, recovery duration, and analgesic consumption. The investigation of a simple, low-cost, pharmacologically active gargling intervention as an adjunct to standard analgesia reflects the spirit of personalized care at the bedside—identifying accessible, evidence-based strategies that may benefit

https://doi.org/10.3390/jpm16050247

specific patient subgroups while minimizing the opioid dependency risk. The rigorous randomized design strengthens the evidentiary value of this contribution.

8. Methodology and Reporting Standards: The Delphi Consensus in Otolaryngology

Underpinning all clinical and translational endeavors in personalized medicine is the quality of the evidence and consensus processes that guide them. The systematic review assessing the reliability and reporting completeness of Delphi consensus studies in otolaryngology addresses a methodological dimension that is of critical importance (Contribution 11). Delphi methodology is increasingly deployed in our specialty to formalize expert agreement in areas where randomized evidence is sparse—precisely the conditions that often characterize emerging personalized medicine interventions. The identification of heterogeneity in reporting standards and the proposal of quality benchmarks represent a significant contribution to the methodological rigor of the field, ensuring that future consensus statements—such as those included in this Special Issue—are held to transparent and reproducible standards.

9. Synthesis and Outlook

Taken together, the eleven papers assembled in this Special Issue articulate a compelling and multi-dimensional vision of personalized medicine in otolaryngology. Several cross-cutting themes emerge from this collection. First, the importance of biomarker-driven and data-informed stratification is evident across contributions ranging from ENE assessment in head and neck cancer to cardiovascular risk stratification in audiological rehabilitation. The trajectory of the field points unmistakably toward the integration of molecular, genetic, electrophysiological, and digital health data streams into routine clinical workflows. Second, the therapeutic potential of drug repurposing, digital health platforms, and minimally invasive surgical innovation underscores that personalization is not synonymous with complexity or cost. Many of the most promising individualized interventions described in this Special Issue are accessible, scalable, and grounded in established biological rationale. Third, the methodological diversity of contributions—encompassing nationwide epidemiological analyses, randomized controlled trials, systematic reviews, meta-analyses, consensus processes, and basic science characterization studies—reflects the pluralistic evidentiary foundation that personalized medicine requires. No single methodology suffices; rather, it is the convergence of complementary approaches that advances understanding. Fourth, the recurring emphasis on quality of life—from vestibular rehabilitation following cochlear implantation, to tinnitus management, to postoperative pain control—affirms that personalized medicine in otolaryngology is not exclusively about survival or disease eradication, but it is about the restoration and preservation of the full spectrum of human sensory and communicative function.

Looking ahead, the field will be shaped by advances in genomics, proteomics, and microbiomics as applied to head and neck oncology and chronic sinonasal disease; by the maturation of gene and stem cell therapies for hereditary hearing loss and laryngotracheal disorders; and by the integration of artificial intelligence into diagnostic imaging, audiological assessment, and surgical planning. The contributions in this Special Issue represent not an endpoint but a foundation—a demonstration of what rigorous, clinically motivated, and methodologically diverse scholarship can achieve in advancing individualized care for patients across the full breadth of our specialty.

I am deeply grateful to all the authors, reviewers, and editorial colleagues whose intellectual generosity and scientific rigor made this Special Issue possible. It is my sincere hope that the work presented here will serve as both a reference and an inspiration for

https://doi.org/10.3390/jpm1605

the next generation of clinicians and researchers who are committed to the promise of personalized medicine in otolaryngology.

Conflicts of Interest: The author declares no conflict of interest.

List of Contributions:

1. Lin, H.-F.; Hung, S.-H. The Diagnostic Gap Between Clinical and Pathological Extranodal Extension in Head and Neck Cancers: A 5-Year Nationwide Trend Analysis in Taiwan. *J. Pers. Med.* **2026**, *16*, 123. https://doi.org/10.3390/jpm16020123.
2. Rodríguez-Prado, C.; Oishi, N.; Fernández-Vidal, E.; Alba-García, J.R.; Zapater, E. Transoral Cordectomy with Microelectrodes (TOMES) on an Outpatient Basis: Advancing Patient Comfort and Personalized Care Through Predictive Models. *J. Pers. Med.* **2025**, *15*, 465. https://doi.org/10.3390/jpm15100465.
3. Di Cesare, T.; Picciotti, P.M.; Di Nardo, W.; Rodolico, D.; Galli, J. Towards a Personalized Vestibular Assessment in Older Patients with Cochlear Implant. *J. Pers. Med.* **2026**, *16*, 81. https://doi.org/10.3390/jpm16020081.
4. Lee, S.-U.; Park, E. Repurposing SGLT-2 Inhibitors as a Novel Therapeutic Strategy for Treatment-Resistant Meniere's Disease. *J. Pers. Med.* **2025**, *15*, 412. https://doi.org/10.3390/jpm15090412.
5. Fieux, M.; Favier, V.; Sousa Machado, A.; Nourredine, M.; Giroudon, C.; Carsuzaa, F.; Naik, P.P.; the yo-IFOS Group. Endoscopic Sinus Surgery in Frontal Sinus Inverted Papilloma: A Systematic Review. *J. Pers. Med.* **2025**, *15*, 183. https://doi.org/10.3390/jpm15050183.
6. Saibene, A.M.; Nitro, L.; Carsuzaa, F.; Alexandru, M.; Bedarida, V.; Di Bari, M.; Fath, L.; Garcia-Lliberos, A.; Legré, M.; Lobo-Duro, D.; et al. Comprehensive Management of Cocaine-Induced Midline Destructive Lesions: A Young-IfOS Consensus. *J. Pers. Med.* **2025**, *15*, 231. https://doi.org/10.3390/jpm15060231.
7. Sia, E.; Tirelli, G.; Gatto, A.; Mineo, C.A.; Curlin, K.; Abouzari, M. Efficacy of Internet-Based Therapies for Tinnitus: A Systematic Review and Meta-Analysis of Randomized Controlled Trials. *J. Pers. Med.* **2024**, *14*, 813. https://doi.org/10.3390/jpm14080813.
8. Tomida, K.; Lee, S.; Makino, K.; Katayama, O.; Harada, K.; Morikawa, M.; Yamaguchi, R.; Nishijima, C.; Fujii, K.; Misu, Y.; et al. Association between Hearing Aid Use and Cognitive Function in Persons with Hearing Impairment Stratified by Cardiovascular Risk. *J. Pers. Med.* **2024**, *14*, 479. https://doi.org/10.3390/jpm14050479.
9. Puig-Herreros, C.; Sanz, J.L.; Barona-Lleó, L.; Forner, L.; Rosell-Clari, V. The Characterization of Normal Male and Female Voice from Surface Electromyographic Parameters. *J. Pers. Med.* **2024**, *14*, 592. https://doi.org/10.3390/jpm14060592.
10. Windpassinger, M.; Prusak, M.; Gemeiner, J.; Plattner, O.; Janik, S.; Besser, G.; Gstoettner, W.; Xuan, P.; Sessler, D.I.; Ruetzler, K. Pain after Licorice or Sugar-Water Gargling in Patients Recovering from Oropharyngeal Surgery—A Randomized, Double-Blind Trial. *J. Pers. Med.* **2024**, *14*, 1056. https://doi.org/10.3390/jpm14101056.
11. Urbanelli, A.; Pugliese, G.; Bolis, E.; Coccapani, M.; Corti, M.G.; D'Angelo, B.; Lancieri, A.; Maggi, L.; Maniaci, A.; Lechien, J.R.; et al. Delphi Consensus in Otolaryngology: A Systematic Review of Reliability and Reporting Completeness. *J. Pers. Med.* **2025**, *15*, 567. https://doi.org/10.3390/jpm15120567.

ferences

Jameson, J.L.; Longo, D.L. Precision Medicine—Personalized, Problematic, and Promising. *N. Engl. J. Med.* **2015**, *372*, 2229–2234. [CrossRef] [PubMed]

Amin, M.B.; Greene, F.L.; Edge, S.B.; Compton, C.C.; Gershenwald, J.E.; Brookland, R.K.; Meyer, L.; Gress, D.M.; Byrd, D.R.; Winchester, D.P. The Eighth Edition AJCC Cancer Staging Manual: Continuing to build a bridge from a population-based to a more "personalized" approach to cancer staging. *CA Cancer J. Clin.* **2017**, *67*, 93–99. [CrossRef] [PubMed]

Agrawal, Y.; Van de Berg, R.; Wuyts, F.; Walther, L.; Magnusson, M.; Oh, E.; Sharpe, M.; Strupp, M. Presbyvestibulopathy: Diagnostic criteria Consensus document of the classification committee of the Bárány Society. *J Vestib. Res.* **2019**, *29*, 161–170. [CrossRef] [PubMed]

4. Trimarchi, M.; Bussi, M.; Sinico, R.A.; Meroni, P.; Specks, U. Cocaine-induced midline destructive lesions—An autoimm disease? *Autoimmun. Rev.* **2013**, *12*, 496–500. [CrossRef] [PubMed]
5. Abouzari, M.; Goshtasbi, K.; Sarna, B.; Ghavami, Y.; Parker, E.M.; Khosravi, P.; Mostaghni, N.; Jamshidi, S.; Saber, T.; Djali H.R. Adapting Personal Therapies Using a Mobile Application for Tinnitus Rehabilitation: A Preliminary Study. *Ann. C Rhinol. Laryngol.* **2021**, *130*, 571–577. [CrossRef] [PubMed]
6. Goshtasbi, K.; Tawk, K.; Khosravi, P.; Abouzari, M.; Djalilian, H.R. Smartphone-Based Cognitive Behavioral Therapy Customized Sound Therapy for Tinnitus: A Randomized Controlled Trial. *Ann. Otol. Rhinol. Laryngol.* **2025**, *134*, 125– [CrossRef] [PubMed]

https://doi.org/10.3390/jpm1605

Journal of
Personalized Medicine

MDPI

cle

sociation between Hearing Aid Use and Cognitive Function Persons with Hearing Impairment Stratified by ardiovascular Risk

ki Tomida *, Sangyoon Lee, Keitaro Makino, Osamu Katayama, Kenji Harada, Masanori Morikawa, Yamaguchi, Chiharu Nishijima, Kazuya Fujii, Yuka Misu and Hiroyuki Shimada

Department of Preventive Gerontology, Center for Gerontology and Social Science, National Center for Geriatrics and Gerontology, Obu 474-8511, Aichi, Japan
* Correspondence: tomida-k@ncgg.go.jp; Tel.: +81-562-44-5651

Abstract: The purpose of this study was to conduct a cross-sectional analysis of the association between hearing aid use and cognitive decline in community-dwelling older adults with hearing impairment, stratified by cardiovascular risk level. This cross-sectional study covers 1857 hearing-impaired individuals selected among 10,674 community-dwelling older adults ($\geq$65 years of age) in Japan. We investigate the association between hearing aid use and cognitive decline stratified by cardiovascular risk level, by assessing self-reported hearing impairment and hearing aid use, absolute cardiovascular risk, cognitive function, and potential confounding factors. The association between hearing impairment severity and increased cardiovascular risk, and the benefit of hearing aid use in preventing cognitive decline, were examined in a binomial logistic regression analysis, with the presence of cognitive decline as the objective variable. In the low cardiovascular risk group, hearing aid users had a lower odds ratio for decline in executive function than non-users (odds ratio = 0.61, 95% confidence interval: 0.39–0.98). However, there was no significant association between hearing aid use and cognitive decline in the high cardiovascular risk group ($p > 0.05$). Among older adults with hearing impairment, hearing aid use was associated with the maintenance of executive function in individuals of low cardiovascular risk.

Keywords: cardiovascular risk; cognitive function; hearing aid; hearing impairment; older adults

1. Introduction

Age-related hearing impairment is the most common sensory impairment associated with aging, with an estimated 1.57 billion people worldwide with hearing impairment by 2019 [1]. This condition leads to increased disability-adjusted life years, which represent health losses [2]. Hearing impairment has been reported to cause communication difficulties, social isolation, and depression, and has been associated with cognitive decline and dementia [3,4]. A previous study reported that a decrease in the frequency of daily conversation is associated with an elevated risk of developing dementia [5]. The association between dementia and hearing impairment has received significant societal attention in recent years, as hearing impairment has been reported to be the most relevant of the modifiable risk factors for dementia [6]. Hearing impairment has also been reported to be associated with mild cognitive impairment [7]; thus, appropriate countermeasures should be taken as early as possible when people begin to notice hearing impairment

Age-related hearing impairment is a sensorineural hearing impairment, characterized by damage to the areas that perceive sound [8]. The main cause is reported to be age-related damage to the hair cells in the cochlea, resulting in a decrease in their number and loss of auditory hairs [9]. Since hair cells are responsible for detecting and amplifying sound, it has been suggested that, when hair cells are damaged, they are unable to successfully transmit sound information to the brain, leading to cognitive decline [10]. In particular, atherosclerotic diseases such as hypertension, diabetes, and cardiovascular disease are thought to increase microcirculatory disturbances, chronic inflammation, and oxidative stress, which can damage the cochlea and auditory nerve and promote more severe hearing impairment [11]. It has also been reported that subclinical atherosclerosis in midlife is associated with hearing impairment in older adults, suggesting that the prevention and control of carotid atherosclerosis in midlife may have a positive impact on hearing health in older adults [12].

Currently, there is no curative treatment for age-related hearing impairment, and it has been reported that compensating for hearing impairment through the use of hearing aids can help prevent dementia and improve quality of life [13]. Recently, it has been shown that hearing impairment is associated with frailty [14], and preventing and controlling hearing impairment is becoming increasingly important in maintaining physical, mental, and cognitive function. In addition, a longitudinal study investigating the association between hearing impairment and physical function decline made the observation that hearing aid users have greater walking endurance [15]. Therefore, hearing aids can be an important tool for older adults with hearing impairment to maintain an active lifestyle. However, a nationwide survey in Japan suggests that hearing aids are not widely used in Japan compared to the United States and Europe, and that the benefits of hearing aids may not be maximized, because the introduction of hearing aids is considered only after the hearing impairment has become more severe [16]. As noted above, microcirculatory disturbances, such as those caused by cardiovascular disease, can damage the cochlea and auditory nerves and accelerate age-related hearing impairment [17]. In this context, the relationship between hearing aid use and cognitive function in the hearing impaired should be examined for individual conditions, especially in light of the impact of cardiovascular risk.

Therefore, the purpose of this study was to conduct a cross-sectional analysis of the association between hearing aid use and cognitive decline in community-dwelling older adults with hearing impairment, stratified by cardiovascular risk level. We hypothesized that, in Japan, where the introduction of hearing aids tends to be delayed, those at a higher risk for cardiovascular disease would have a more severe hearing impairment, which could reduce the benefits of hearing aid use.

2. Materials and Methods

2.1. Participants

This cross-sectional study involved community-dwelling older Japanese adults ($\geq$65 years of age), who resided in Japan. They were recruited from a sub-cohort of a large cohort study, which aims to identify the risks of geriatric syndromes that occur with aging and to identify effective ways to treat them [18].

Individuals were interviewed regarding their self-report questionnaire assessment of hearing impairment and hearing aid use; those that were not hearing-impaired and those who had deficits in their assessment results were excluded. We then applied the following exclusion criteria: (1) a history of Alzheimer's disease, Parkinson's disease, or stroke; (2) impairment in basic activities of daily living (ADLs); (3) needing support and care by the long-term care insurance (LTCI) system at the time of assessment; (4) severe cognitive impairment (Mini-Mental State Examination [MMSE] score $\leqq$ 21); and (5) missing data of exclusion criteria. Participants were evaluated by medical history assessments, sociodemographic information, blood sampling, and physical activity measurements.

The health check-up survey was undertaken by well-trained nurses and study assistants in community centers. All staff received training from the authors in terms of the protocols for administering the assessments prior to study commencement.

2.2. Ethical Approval

This study was conducted in accordance with the principles of the Declaration of Helsinki. The study protocol was approved by the Ethics Committee of the National Center for Geriatrics and Gerontology (approval number: 1440-5). Written informed consent was obtained from all participants before their inclusion in the study.

2.3. *Measures*

2.3.1. Assessment of Self-Reported Hearing Impairment and Hearing Aid Use

Prior to the start of the study, the authors trained staff on the protocols for administering participant assessments. During these assessments, nurses asked participants whether they used hearing aids on a daily basis.

Participants also completed the Hearing Handicap Inventory for the Elderly Screening Version (HHIE-S) [19]. The HHIE-S questionnaire measures activity and participation restrictions caused by hearing impairment in various situations of daily life. The 10 items of the HHIE-S are classified into two subscales: one exploring emotional consequences, and another exploring social or situational effects. Each item has three response options: "yes" (score = 4), "sometimes" (2), and "no" (0). Hearing aid users and those with a total HHIE-S score greater than 8 were classified as having a hearing impairment [19].

2.3.2. Estimation of Absolute Cardiovascular Risk

The revised WHO risk estimation chart was used to evaluate 10-year cardiovascular disease risk [20]. This chart shows the absolute risk of cardiovascular disease events according to an individual's risk status, with higher risk scores indicating a greater burden of risk factors. The development group calibrated the prediction model for 21 regions of the world, with region-specific prediction charts. Two types of prediction tables are available: laboratory-based models that include medical history and blood data, and non-laboratory-based models consisting of convenient variables in resource-limited settings. In this study, we used a laboratory-based risk estimation model including age, sex, a history of diabetes, smoking status, systolic blood pressure, and total cholesterol for a high-income Asia–Pacific region, including Japan [20].

A current history of diabetes was assessed during a face-to-face interview with a nurse. The nurse measured systolic blood pressure using an automated blood pressure monitor, while the participant was seated. Serum total cholesterol levels (in mmol/L) were measured by the cholesterol oxidative enzymatic (COD-POD) method in a laboratory (SRL, Inc., Japan, Tokyo). Smoking status (smoked regularly, current vs. former/never) was assessed by the research assistants. Finally, we calculated absolute cardiovascular risk (%), based on the above risk status, using the revised WHO risk estimation charts and stratified cardiovascular risk levels, namely, low ($\leq$20%) and high ($\geq$20%).

2.3.3. Measurements of Cognitive Function

Cognitive function was assessed using the National Center for Geriatrics and Gerontology–Functional Assessment Tool (NCGG-FAT) [21,22], which was administered by well-trained staff using appropriate testing protocols. The primary outcomes included four cognitive domain tests: memory (word list memory-I [immediate recognition], word list memory-II [delayed recognition]), attention (electronic tablet version of the Trail Making Test [TMT] Part A), executive function (electronic tablet version of the TMT Part B), and processing speed (electronic tablet version of the Symbolic Digit Substitution Test). The NCGG-FAT has been found to have high test–retest reliability and moderate-to-high validity among community-dwelling older adults [21]. All the tests have established standardized thresholds for defining objective cognitive impairment in the corresponding domains (a score of $\geq$1.5 standard deviations [SD] below the age- and education-specific means, based on an algorithm obtained from a database including over 10,000 community-dwelling older adults), which were derived from a population-based cohort [23].

2.3.4. Potential Confounding Factors

Potential confounders of dementia and hearing impairment included age, gender, body mass index (BMI), years of education, and exercise habits [6]. The BMI was calculated using height and weight and measured using a bioelectrical impedance analyzer (Tanita MC780A; Tanita Corporation, Tokyo, Japan) [24]. To assess exercise habits, participants were asked, "Do you exercise moderately for your health?" and participants who answered "no" were considered physically inactive. Otherwise, depression was assessed using the 15-item Geriatric Depression Scale (GDS) [25]. A cutoff score of 6 or higher has an 82% sensitivity and 75% specificity in a structured clinical interview for depression [26]. Cognitive functioning was assessed using the Mini-Mental State Examination (MMSE) [27,28].

2.4. Statistical Analysis

Baseline characteristics were compared according to cardiovascular risk levels (low- and high-risk levels), using the unpaired *t*-test for continuous variables and a $\chi 2$ test for categorical variables.

To examine the association between hearing aid use and cognitive function, a binomial logistic regression analysis was performed in the presence or absence of functional decline in each cognitive domain as the objective variable. This model was applied to the overall sample and to the cardiovascular-risk-level-stratified sample (low and high risk). In these models, odds ratios (ORs) and 95% confidence intervals (CIs) for cognitive function were calculated in crude and adjusted models, using hearing aid use as the explanatory variable. Adjusted models were adjusted for the following potential confounding factors: age, sex, BMI, educational level, and exercise habits. Analyses were conducted using IBM SPSS Statistics software package version 27.0 (SPSS Corp., Armonk, NY, USA). The level of statistical significance was set a priori at $p < 0.05$.

3. Results

3.1. Participants

Among the 10,674 individuals that participated in the health check-up survey, 2330 were hearing-impaired and, therefore, pre-selected for the study. After exclusion criteria were applied, 1857 individuals were enrolled (Figure 1). Data for analysis were obtained from medical history and sociodemographic information, blood sampling, and physical activity measurements.

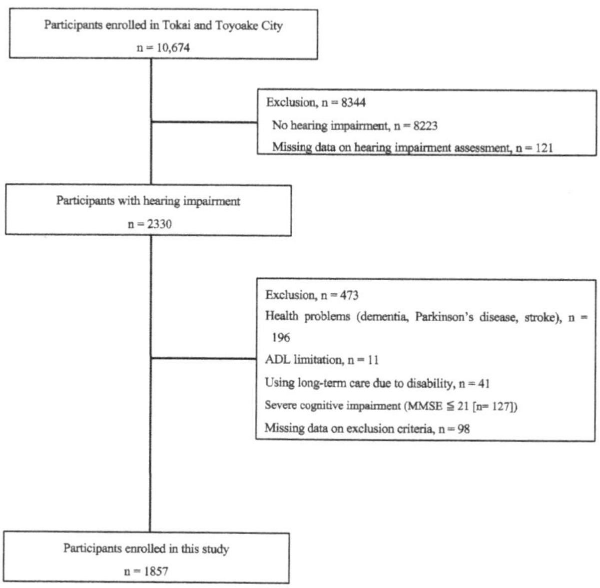

Figure 1. Flowchart of sample selection.

3.2. Characteristics of Hearing Impaired by Estimated Cardiovascular Risk Level

Among the 1857 participants with hearing impairment, 985 (53.0%) were allocated to the cardiovascular low-risk group and 872 (47.0%) were allocated to the high-risk group. The differences in participant characteristics between the two cardiovascular risk groups are shown in Table 1. Significant differences were found in all components of the WHO risk estimation model: age ($p < 0.001$), sex ($p < 0.001$), diabetes prevalence ($p < 0.001$), percentage of current smokers ($p < 0.001$), systolic blood pressure ($p < 0.001$), and total cholesterol ($p < 0.001$). In addition, there were significant differences between cardiovascular risk levels in BMI ($p < 0.001$), education level ($p = 0.038$), and hearing aid use ($p = 0.014$). There were no significant differences in history of depression, HHIE-S scores, MMSE scores, and exercise habits ($p > 0.05$).

Table 1. Characteristics of hearing-impaired participants stratified by estimated cardiovascular risk level.

		Overall n = 1857	Cardiovascular Risk Levels		*p*
			Low-Risk Group (<20%) n = 985 (53.0%)	High-Risk Group (≧20%) n = 872 (47.0%)	
Age	years	76.1 ± 6.0	75.1 ± 6.2	77.3 ± 5.6	<0.001 [a]
Sex, female	n (%)	875 (47.1)	568 (57.7) [c]	307 (35.2) [d]	<0.001 [b]
Diabetes mellitus, yes	n (%)	260 (14.0)	24 (2.4) [d]	236 (27.1) [c]	<0.001 [b]
Smoking status, yes	n (%)	142 (7.6)	120 (12.2) [c]	22 (2.5) [d]	<0.001 [b]
Systolic blood pressure	mmHg	145.1 ± 19.6	134.3 ± 15.6	157.3 ± 16.3	<0.001 [a]
Total cholesterol	mmol/l	5.3 ± 0.9	5.2 ± 0.8	5.4 ± 0.9	<0.001 [a]
BMI	point	23.1 ± 3.1	22.8 ± 3.2	23.4 ± 2.9	<0.001 [a]
Depression, yes	n (%)	37 (2.0)	24 (2.4)	13 (1.5)	0.146 [b]
Education level	years	11.5 ± 2.4	11.6 ± 2.4	11.3 ± 2.4	0.038 [a]
MMSE	score	26.7 ± 2.3	26.8 ± 2.3	26.6 ± 2.3	0.059 [a]
HHIE-S	score	16.8 ± 8.0	16.5 ± 7.9	17.2 ± 8.1	0.073 [a]
Hearing aid use, yes	n (%)	454 (24.4)	218 (22.1) [d]	236 (27.1) [c]	0.014 [b]
Exercise habits, yes	n (%)	563 (30.3)	306 (31.1)	257 (29.5)	0.456 [b]

BMI, Body mass index; MMSE, Mini-Mental State Examination; HHIE-S, Hearing Handicap Inventory for the Elderly–Screening. Data are expressed as mean ± standard deviation or numbers (%). [a] = *p*-values reported from unpaired *t*-test. [b] = *p*-values obtained by Pearson's chi-squared test. [c] = Statistically significant association by adjusted standardized residual > 1.96 [$p < 0.05$]. [d] = Statistically significant association by adjusted standardized residual < −1.96 [$p < 0.05$].

3.3. Associations between Hearing Aid Use and Cognitive Function

Table 2 presents the results of the binomial logistic regression analysis for the total sample (n = 1857), the presence of a functional decline in each cognitive domain as the objective variable, and hearing aid use as the explanatory variable.

Table 2. Binomial logistic regression results showing associations between hearing aid use and cognitive function.

Cognitive Function	Variables	Crude Model		Adjusted Model	
		OR (95% CI)	*p*-Value	OR (95% CI)	*p*-Value
Memory (Score < 1.5SD), yes	Hearing aid user	0.88 (0.59–1.31)	0.526	0.94 (0.62–1.42)	0.771
	Age			0.98 (0.95–1.01)	0.180
	Sex, female			0.60 (0.42–0.85)	0.004
	BMI			1.00 (0.95–1.06)	0.954
	Education level			0.91 (0.84–0.98)	0.015
	Exercise habits			0.63 (0.42–0.95)	0.028
Attention (Time < 1.5SD), yes	Hearing aid user	0.92 (0.59–1.42)	0.691	0.94 (0.62–1.42)	0.601
	Age			1.01 (0.98–1.04)	0.537
	Sex, female			0.85 (0.59–1.24)	0.408

Table 2. *Cont.*

Cognitive Function	Variables	Crude Model		Adjusted Model	
		OR (95% CI)	*p*-Value	OR (95% CI)	*p*-Value
	BMI			1.00 (0.95–1.07)	0.906
	Education level			0.95 (0.87–1.03)	0.182
	Exercise habits, yes			0.59 (0.38–0.94)	0.025
Executive function (Time < 1.5SD), yes	Hearing aid user	0.93 (0.69–1.25)	0.615	0.76 (0.55–1.03)	0.075
	Age			1.07 (1.05–1.10)	<0.001
	Sex, female			1.15 (0.89–1.50)	0.279
	BMI			1.02 (0.98–1.06)	0.359
	Education level			0.88 (0.83–0.93)	<0.001
	Exercise habits, yes			0.65 (0.47–0.88)	0.005
Processing speed (Score < 1.5SD), yes	Hearing aid user	0.75 (0.37–1.51)	0.416	0.71 (0.35–1.46)	0.357
	Age			1.02 (0.97–1.07)	0.430
	Sex, female			0.90 (0.51–1.59)	0.718
	BMI			1.02 (0.93–1.11)	0.744
	Education level			0.90 (0.79–1.02)	0.092
	Exercise habits, yes			1.04 (0.56–1.93)	0.910

In both the crude and adjusted models, there was no significant association between hearing aid use and cognitive function for functional decline in each cognitive domain (memory, attention, executive function, and processing speed) ($p > 0.05$).

3.4. Associations between Hearing Aid Use and Cognitive Function Stratified by Cardiovascular Risk Levels

The results of the binomial logistic regression analysis in the cardiovascular-risk-level-stratified sample are shown in Table 3. In the low cardiovascular risk group (n = 985), there was an association between hearing aid use and cognitive function in persons with hearing impairment in the cognitive domain of executive function (OR, 0.61; 95% CI: 0.39–0.98; $p = 0.039$). However, no other statistically significant associations with cognitive function were detected. In the high cardiovascular risk group (n = 872), the association between hearing aid use and cognitive function in persons with hearing loss was not significant with any cognitive function ($p > 0.05$).

Table 3. Binomial logistic regression showing associations between hearing aid use and cognitive function, stratified by absolute cardiovascular risk levels.

Cognitive Function	Variables	Cardiovascular Risk Levels			
		Low-Risk Group (<20%)		High-Risk Group (≧20%)	
		OR (95% CI)	*p*-Value	OR (95% CI)	*p*-Value
Memory (Score < 1.5SD), yes	Hearing aid user	0.86 (0.49–1.54)	0.621	1.04 (0.57–1.89)	0.910
	Age	0.98 (0.94–1.01)	0.213	1.00 (0.95–1.05)	0.966
	Sex, female	0.59 (0.38–0.93)	0.024	0.48 (0.26–0.89)	0.019
	BMI	0.96 (0.89–1.03)	0.221	1.08 (0.99–1.18)	0.080
	Education level	0.90 (0.81–0.99)	0.038	0.92 (0.82–1.04)	0.168
	Exercise habits, yes	0.62 (0.36–1.06)	0.082	0.68 (0.36–1.30)	0.216
	BMI	0.96 (0.89–1.03)	0.221	1.08 (0.99–1.18)	0.080
	Education level	0.90 (0.81–0.99)	0.038	0.92 (0.82–1.04)	0.168
	Exercise habits, yes	0.62 (0.36–1.06)	0.082	0.68 (0.36–1.30)	0.216
Attention (Time < 1.5SD), yes	Hearing aid user	0.87 (0.47–1.61)	0.653	0.93 (0.49–1.79)	0.831
	Age	1.02 (0.98–1.06)	0.400	1.01 (0.95–1.06)	0.860
	Sex, female	0.67 (0.40–1.10)	0.111	1.06 (0.59–1.89)	0.844
	BMI	1.00 (0.92–1.08)	0.937	1.02 (0.93–1.12)	0.735
	Education level	0.94 (0.84–1.05)	0.248	0.95 (0.83–1.08)	0.400
	Exercise habits, yes	0.69 (0.39–1.24)	0.219	0.49 (0.23–1.03)	0.058

Table 3. *Cont.*

Cognitive Function	Variables	Cardiovascular Risk Levels			
		Low-Risk Group (<20%)		High-Risk Group (≧20%)	
		OR (95% CI)	*p*-Value	OR (95% CI)	*p*-Value
ecutive function (Time < 1.5SD), yes	Hearing aid user	0.61 (0.39–0.98)	0.039	0.93 (0.61–1.42)	0.740
	Age	1.08 (1.05–1.11)	<0.001	1.07 (1.03–1.11)	<0.001
	Sex, female	0.93 (0.65–1.34)	0.698	1.33 (0.91–1.95)	0.141
	BMI	1.02 (0.96–1.08)	0.526	1.02 (0.96–1.09)	0.515
	Education level	0.84 (0.77–0.91)	<0.001	0.92 (0.84–1.00)	0.047
	Exercise habits, yes	0.65 (0.42–0.99)	0.045	0.66 (0.42–1.04)	0.070
ocessing speed (Score < 1.5SD), yes	Hearing aid user	0.67 (0.25–1.80)	0.424	0.81 (0.28–2.29)	0.688
	Age	1.04 (0.98–1.11)	0.205	1.00 (0.92–1.08)	0.898
	Sex, female	0.78 (0.37–1.70)	0.526	0.88 (0.35–2.19)	0.777
	BMI	0.94 (0.83–1.07)	0.338	1.12 (0.98–1.28)	0.108
	Education level	0.78 (0.65–0.93)	0.007	1.04 (0.87–1.25)	0.677
	Exercise habits, yes	1.48 (0.67–3.30)	0.337	0.68 (0.25–1.89)	0.464

4. Discussion

This cross-sectional study used a logistic regression analysis with data from 1857 community-dwelling older adults with a hearing impairment, stratified by cardiovascular risk level, to determine associations between hearing aid use and the function of cognitive function. The result, a stratified analysis by cardiovascular risk level, showed no association between hearing aid use and the function of cognitive function in the high-risk group. This association, however, was found in the cardiovascular low-risk-level group. A possible explanation for this discrepancy is that high cardiovascular risk levels may adversely affect the progression of hearing impairment, possibly overriding the benefit of hearing aid use. As shown in Table 1, the group at higher cardiovascular risk has more people with diabetes, a smoking habit, higher blood pressure and total cholesterol levels, and a significantly higher BMI than the group at a lower cardiovascular risk. The number of hearing aid users is also significantly higher in the high cardiovascular risk group. The results emphasize the importance of introducing hearing aids before the hearing impairment becomes more severe and maintaining a lifestyle that keeps the level of cardiovascular risk low, in order to maximize the benefits of hearing aids.

Currently, there is no definitive cure for dementia, and attempts are being made to develop a variety of preventive interventions and treatments to delay its onset and progression. Hearing impairment has been reported as a relevant risk factor for dementia [6]. It has been suggested that hearing impairment limits the activities of daily living and narrows the life space [29] and may make it difficult to maintain an active lifestyle, which is important for dementia prevention [29]. Furthermore, it has been reported that the risk of nursing care is 1.7 times higher for those with hearing impairment, when accompanied by a feeling of loneliness [30]. In Japan, dementia is the leading cause of the need for nursing care [31], and appropriate care for hearing impairment may lead to the prevention of dementia and the need for nursing care. Indeed, early intervention with the use of hearing aids has been reported to prevent the onset of dementia and the progression of its symptoms [13]. However, the mechanisms linking hearing impairment and dementia have not been elucidated, and it remains unclear how hearing impairment affects various cognitive domains. This study showed an association between hearing aid use and a reduced decline in executive function in community-dwelling older adults with hearing impairment and low levels of cardiovascular risk. Executive function represents cognitive and intellectual abilities controlled by the frontal lobes, which are considered higher in the cognitive hierarchy than cognitive domains such as memory, perception, language, etc. [32]. Executive dysfunction has also been reported to be associated with depression, and the clinical features of depression and frontal lobe disorders are thought to be similar [33]. Age-related hearing impairment has been associated with depression and has been linked to cognitive decline and dementia [34]. Thus, in individuals with hearing impairment, it may promote a decline in executive function, which is regulated by frontal lobe function.

Age-related hearing impairment is a sensorineural hearing impairment caused by age-related damage to the outer hair cells of the cochlea and a decrease in the number of cells [34]. Recent evidence indicates that reactive oxygen species are involved in the development of hearing impairment [35]. Previous studies have shown that age-related hearing impairment is accelerated by microcirculatory disturbances, chronic inflammation, oxidative stress, and cardiovascular disease [11]. It has also been reported that subclinical atherosclerosis in midlife is associated with hearing impairment in older adults [12]. These findings suggest that, when cardiovascular risk is high, microcirculatory impairment, chronic inflammation, and oxidative stress accelerate the cell death of outer hair cells in the inner ear, the cause of age-related hearing impairment, resulting in a more severe hearing impairment. As an effective countermeasure for these problems, it has been suggested that increasing physical activity through exercise may promote antioxidant activity and help prevent hearing impairment [36]. However, sufficient evidence has not yet been obtained to verify whether exercise contributes to the improvement of hearing impairment or to the maintenance of hearing function. Therefore, the introduction of hearing aids is considered to be the first choice for hearing impairment, and it is increasingly important to establish the timing of their introduction and appropriate evaluation methods.

This study is a large-cohort study of community-dwelling older adults with hearing impairment. Although a number of cardiovascular risks have been reported to be associated with hearing impairment, their impact on hearing aid use has not been fully explored. Therefore, we consider this study to provide a baseline for further research. However, there are several limitations to this study. First, the participants' hearing tests were based on self-report questionnaires and did not use objective measures. Also, because this is a cross-sectional study, it is unclear whether hearing aid use contributed to cognitive function in a causal manner. In addition, another limitation is the lack of information about when participants started using hearing aids, their compliance and degree of hearing impairment, the character of their hearing problems, and the duration of their hearing impairment. In future studies, we would like to add objective assessments to the hearing screening, and analyze the effects of hearing aid use on cognitive function longitudinally to examine the relationship between hearing impairment and cognitive function in more detail.

5. Conclusions

The association between hearing aid use and cognitive function, stratified by cardiovascular risk level, was investigated in a cross-sectional analysis of community-dwelling older adults with hearing impairment. Among older adults with a hearing impairment, hearing aid use was associated with the maintenance of executive function in individuals of low cardiovascular risk. Increased cardiovascular risk level may promote arteriosclerotic, and increase the severity of sensorineural, hearing impairment. These results suggest that it is important to consider hearing aid use even before hearing impairment becomes severe, to keep the cardiovascular disease risk level low and to maintain lifestyle habits that limit inner ear dysfunction. Further verification is required to determine what effect the use of hearing aids has on the health status of older adults, including the prevention of cognitive decline.

Author Contributions: K.T. was responsible for the following contributor roles; Conceptualization, Data curation, Formal analysis, Funding acquisition, Investigation, Methodology, and Writing—original draft. S.L., K.M., O.K. and K.H. were responsible for the following contributor roles; Investigation, Methodology, Resources, Software, and Writing—review & editing. M.M., R.Y., C.N., K.F. and Y.M. were responsible for the following contributor roles; Data curation, Formal analysis, Validation, Investigation, Methodology, Resources, Software, and Writing—review & editing. H.S., was responsible for the following contributor roles; Funding acquisition, Project administrarion, Supervision, and Writing—review & editing. All authors have read and agreed to the published version of the manuscript.

Funding: This work received financial support via AMED (18dk0110021h0003, 18le0110004h0002), Research Funding for Longevity Sciences from the National Center for Geriatrics and Gerontology (27-22), JSPS KAKENHI Grant in Aid of Scientific Research Activity start-ups (21K21183), and Grant in Aid of Young Scientists (23K16666). No support was received from private industry. The funding sources played no role in the design or conduct of the study; collection, management, analysis, or interpretation of the data; or preparation, review, or approval of the manuscript.

Institutional Review Board Statement: The study protocol was approved by the Ethics Committee of the National Center for Geriatrics and Gerontology (approval number: 1440-5). This study was conducted in accordance with the principles of the Declaration of Helsinki.

Informed Consent Statement: Written informed consent was obtained from all participants before their inclusion in the study.

Data Availability Statement: The datasets used and/or analyzed during the present study are available from the corresponding author upon reasonable request.

Conflicts of Interest: The authors declare that there are no conflicts of interest. The funders had no role in the design of the study; in the collection, analyses, or interpretation of data; in the writing of the manuscript; or in the decision to publish the results.

erences

Haile, L.M.; Kamenov, K.; Briant, P.S.; Orji, A.U.; Steinmetz, J.D.; Abdoli, A.; Abdollahi, M.; Abu-Gharbieh, E.; Afshin, A.; Ahmed, H.; et al. Hearing loss prevalence and years lived with disability, 1990–2019: Findings from the Global Burden of Disease Study 2019. *Lancet* **2021**, *397*, 996–1009. [CrossRef] [PubMed]
Vos, T. Global burden of 369 diseases and injuries in 204 countries and territories, 1990–2019: A systematic analysis for the Global Burden of Disease Study 2019. *Lancet* **2020**, *396*, 1204–1222. [CrossRef] [PubMed]
Shukla, A.; Harper, M.; Pedersen, E.; Goman, A.; Suen, J.J.; Price, C.; Applebaum, J.; Hoyer, M.; Lin, F.R.; Reed, N.S. Hearing Loss, Loneliness, and Social Isolation: A Systematic Review. *Otolaryngol. Head Neck Surg.* **2020**, *162*, 622–633. [CrossRef] [PubMed]
Rutherford, B.R.; Brewster, K.; Golub, J.S.; Kim, A.H.; Roose, S.P. Sensation and Psychiatry: Linking Age-Related Hearing Loss to Late-Life Depression and Cognitive Decline. *Am. J. Psychiatry* **2018**, *175*, 215–224. [CrossRef] [PubMed]
Shimada, H.; Doi, T.; Tsutsumimoto, K.; Makino, K.; Harada, K.; Tomida, K.; Arai, H. Elevated Risk of Dementia Diagnosis in Older Adults with Low Frequencies and Durations of Social Conversation. *J. Alzheimer's Dis.* **2024**, *98*, 659–669. [CrossRef]
Livingston, G.; Huntley, J.; Sommerlad, A.; Ames, D.; Ballard, C.; Banerjee, S.; Brayne, C.; Burns, A.; Cohen-Mansfield, J.; Cooper, C.; et al. Dementia prevention, intervention, and care: 2020 report of the Lancet Commission. *Lancet* **2020**, *396*, 413–446. [CrossRef]
Tomida, K.; Lee, S.; Bae, S.; Harada, K.; Katayama, O.; Makino, K.; Chiba, I.; Morikawa, M.; Shimada, H. Association of Dual Sensory Impairment with Cognitive Decline in Older Adults. *Dement. Geriatr. Cogn. Disord.* **2022**, *51*, 322–330. [CrossRef] [PubMed]
Bowl, M.R.; Dawson, S.J. Age-Related Hearing Loss. *Cold Spring Harb. Perspect. Med.* **2019**, *9*, a033217. [CrossRef] [PubMed]
Liberman, M.C.; Kujawa, S.G. Cochlear synaptopathy in acquired sensorineural hearing loss: Manifestations and mechanisms. *Hear. Res.* **2017**, *349*, 138–147. [CrossRef]
Slade, K.; Plack, C.J.; Nuttall, H.E. The Effects of Age-Related Hearing Loss on the Brain and Cognitive Function. *Trends Neurosci.* **2020**, *43*, 810–821. [CrossRef]
Yamasoba, T.; Lin, F.R.; Someya, S.; Kashio, A.; Sakamoto, T.; Kondo, K. Current concepts in age-related hearing loss: Epidemiology and mechanistic pathways. *Hear. Res.* **2013**, *303*, 30–38. [CrossRef]
Morales, E.E.; Croll, P.H.; Palta, P.; Goedegebure, A.; Reed, N.S.; Betz, J.F.; Lin, F.R.; Deal, J.A. Association of Carotid Atherosclerosis With Hearing Loss: A Cross-sectional Analysis of the Atherosclerosis Risk in Communities Study. *JAMA Otolaryngol. Head Neck Surg.* **2023**, *149*, 223–230. [CrossRef]
Yeo, B.S.; Song, H.J.; Toh, E.M.; Ng, L.S.; Ho, C.S.; Ho, R.; Merchant, R.A.; Tan, B.K.; Loh, W.S. Association of Hearing Aids and Cochlear Implants With Cognitive Decline and Dementia: A Systematic Review and Meta-analysis. *JAMA Neurol.* **2023**, *80*, 134–141. [CrossRef] [PubMed]
Tan, B.K.J.; Man, R.E.K.; Gan, A.T.L.; Fenwick, E.K.; Varadaraj, V.; Swenor, B.K.; Gupta, P.; Wong, T.Y.; Trevisan, C.; Lorenzo-López, L.; et al. Is Sensory Loss an Understudied Risk Factor for Frailty? A Systematic Review and Meta-analysis. *J. Gerontol. A Biol. Sci. Med. Sci.* **2020**, *75*, 2461–2470. [CrossRef]
Martinez-Amezcua, P.; Kuo, P.-L.; Reed, N.S.; Simonsick, E.M.; Agrawal, Y.; Lin, F.R.; Deal, J.A.; Ferrucci, L.; Schrack, J.A. Association of Hearing Impairment With Higher-Level Physical Functioning and Walking Endurance: Results From the Baltimore Longitudinal Study of Aging. *J. Gerontol. A Biol. Sci. Med. Sci.* **2021**, *76*, e290–e298. [CrossRef] [PubMed]
Japan Hearing Aid Manufacturers Association. *JAPAN Trak 2022 Report*; Japan Hearing Aid Manufacturers Association: Japan, Tokyo, 2022.
Kakarlapudi, V.; Sawyer, R.; Staecker, H. The effect of diabetes on sensorineural hearing loss. *Otol. Neurotol.* **2003**, *24*, 382–386. [CrossRef]

18. Shimada, H.; Tsutsumimoto, K.; Lee, S.; Doi, T.; Makizako, H.; Lee, S.; Harada, K.; Hotta, R.; Bae, S.; Nakakubo, S.; et al. Driv continuity in cognitively impaired older drivers. *Geriatr. Gerontol. Int.* **2016**, *16*, 508–514. [CrossRef] [PubMed]
19. Tomioka, K.; Ikeda, H.; Hanaie, K.; Morikawa, M.; Iwamoto, J.; Okamoto, N.; Saeki, K.; Kurumatani, N. The Hearing Hand Inventory for Elderly-Screening (HHIE-S) versus a single question: Reliability, validity, and relations with quality of life meas in the elderly community, Japan. *Qual. Life Res.* **2013**, *22*, 1151–1159. [CrossRef]
20. Kaptoge, S.; Pennells, L.; De Bacquer, D.; Cooney, M.T.; Kavousi, M.; Stevens, G.; Riley, L.M.; Savin, S.; Khan, T.; Altay, S.; World Health Organization cardiovascular disease risk charts: Revised models to estimate risk in 21 global regions. *Lancet C Health* **2019**, *7*, e1332–e1345. [CrossRef]
21. Makizako, H.; Shimada, H.; Park, H.; Doi, T.; Yoshida, D.; Uemura, K.; Tsutsumimoto, K.; Suzuki, T. Evaluation of multidin sional neurocognitive function using a tablet personal computer: Test–retest reliability and validity in community-dwelling o adults. *Geriatr. Gerontol. Int.* **2013**, *13*, 860–866. [CrossRef]
22. Shimada, H.; Makizako, H.; Park, H.; Doi, T.; Lee, S. Validity of the National Center for Geriatrics and Gerontology-Functi Assessment Tool and Mini-Mental State Examination for detecting the incidence of dementia in older Japanese adults. *Ger Gerontol. Int.* **2017**, *17*, 2383–2388. [CrossRef] [PubMed]
23. Shimada, H.; Makizako, H.; Doi, T.; Yoshida, D.; Tsutsumimoto, K.; Anan, Y.; Uemura, K.; Ito, T.; Lee, S.; Park, H.; et al. Combi prevalence of frailty and mild cognitive impairment in a population of elderly Japanese people. *J. Am. Med. Dir. Assoc.* **2013** 518–524. [CrossRef] [PubMed]
24. Nuñez, C.; Gallagher, D.; Visser, M.; Pi-Sunyer, F.X.; Wang, Z.; Heymsfield, S.B. Bioimpedance analysis: Evaluation of leg-to system based on pressure contact footpad electrodes. *Med. Sci. Sports Exerc.* **1997**, *29*, 524–531. [CrossRef] [PubMed]
25. Yesavage, J.A.; Brink, T.L.; Rose, T.L.; Lum, O.; Huang, V.; Adey, M.; Leirer, V.O. Development and validation of a geria depression screening scale: A preliminary report. *J. Psychiatr. Res.* **1982**, *17*, 37–49. [CrossRef] [PubMed]
26. Friedman, B.; Heisel, M.J.; Delavan, R.L. Psychometric properties of the 15-item geriatric depression scale in function impaired, cognitively intact, community-dwelling elderly primary care patients. *J. Am. Geriatr. Soc.* **2005**, *53*, 1570–1 [CrossRef] [PubMed]
27. Folestein, M.F.; Mchugh, P.R. "Mini-mental state". A practical method for grading the cognitive state of patients for the clini *J. Psychiat. Res.* **1975**, *12*, 189–198.
28. Tsoi, K.K.; Chan, J.Y.; Hirai, H.W.; Wong, S.Y.; Kwok, T.C. Cognitive Tests to Detect Dementia: A Systematic Review Meta-analysis. *JAMA Intern. Med.* **2015**, *175*, 1450–1458. [CrossRef] [PubMed]
29. Tomida, K.; Lee, S.; Bae, S.; Makino, K.; Chiba, I.; Harada, K.; Katayama, O.; Morikawa, M.; Shimada, H. Association of c sensory impairment with changes in life space: A longitudinal study with two-year follow-up. *Maturitas* **2022**, *165*, 78 [CrossRef] [PubMed]
30. Tomida, K.; Lee, S.; Makino, K.; Katayama, O.; Harada, K.; Morikawa, M.; Yamaguchi, R.; Nishijima, C.; Fujii, K.; Misu, Y.; e Association of Loneliness With the Incidence of Disability in Older Adults With Hearing Impairment in Japan. *JAMA Otolary Neck Surg.* **2023**, *149*, 439–446. [CrossRef]
31. Ministry of Health, Labour and Welfare. *Summary of the 2019 National Survey of Basic Living Conditions in Japan*; Ministry of He Labour and Welfare: Tokyo, Japan, 2019.
32. Mulrow, C.D.; Aguilar, C.; Endicott, J.E.; Tuley, M.R.; Velez, R.; Charlip, W.S.; Rhodes, M.C.; Hill, J.A.; DeNino, L.A. Quality-of changes and hearing impairment. A randomized trial. *Ann. Intern. Med.* **1990**, *113*, 188–194. [CrossRef]
33. Friedman, N.P.; Robbins, T.W. The role of prefrontal cortex in cognitive control and executive function. *Neuropsychopharmaco* **2022**, *47*, 72–89. [CrossRef] [PubMed]
34. Ciorba, A.; Bianchini, C.; Pelucchi, S.; Pastore, A. The impact of hearing loss on the quality of life of elderly adults. *Clin. In Aging* **2012**, *7*, 159–163. [CrossRef] [PubMed]
35. Lockwood, K.A.; Alexopoulos, G.S.; van Gorp, W.G. Executive dysfunction in geriatric depression. *Am. J. Psychiatry* **2002**, 1119–1126. [CrossRef] [PubMed]
36. Oishi, T.; Matsumaru, D.; Ota, N.; Kitamura, H.; Zhang, T.; Honkura, Y.; Katori, Y.; Motohashi, H. Activation of the NRF2 path in Keap1-knockdown mice attenuates progression of age-related hearing loss. *npj Aging Mech. Dis.* **2020**, *6*, 14. [Cross [PubMed]

Journal of
Personalized
Medicine

MDPI

cle

ıe Characterization of Normal Male and Female Voice from ırface Electromyographic Parameters

ra Puig-Herreros [1], José Luis Sanz [2,*], Luz Barona-Lleó [3], Leopoldo Forner [2] and Vicent Rosell-Clari [1]

[1] Speech Therapy University Clinic, Department of Basic Psychology, Universitat de València, Avda. de Blasco Ibáñez, 21, 46010 Valencia, Spain
[2] Department of Stomatology, Faculty of Medicine and Dentistry, Universitat de València, C/Gascó Oliag 1, 46010 Valencia, Spain
[3] Department of Otolaryngology, Barona Clinic, "Casa de Salud" Hospital, Calle Manuel Candela, 41, 46021 Valencia, Spain
* Correspondence: jose.l.sanz@uv.es

Abstract: Currently, there is no consensus on the characterization of the human voice. The objective of the present study is to describe the myoelectric behavior of the extrinsic musculature of the larynx in 146 people with normal voice (Spanish speakers), aged between 20 and 50 years old. Different vocal tasks were recorded using a surface electromyograph (SEMG). In all vocal tasks, it was observed that women had higher activation (μV) in the suprahyoid and sternocleidomastoid muscles than men, while men had higher activation in the infrahyoid muscles. SEMG is a valid procedure to help define normal vocal characteristics in the studied population, providing reference values during clinical examination. However, it is necessary to adopt a universal system of assessment tasks and standardized measurement techniques to allow for comparisons with future studies.

Keywords: voice; characterization; surface electromyography

1. Introduction

Among the procedures for the study of muscle electrical activity are electromyography (EMG) and surface electromyography (SEMG). The former analyzes and records the myoelectric activity of muscle fibers for the diagnosis of neuromuscular diseases, using needle insertion [1]. SEMG uses surface electrodes, one of which serves as a reference (neutral electrode) located in the vicinity of electrically inactive tissue such as bones or tendons, for example, in our case, as will be described below, in the olecranon, in order to avoid interference.

Surface electromyography (SEMG) records myoelectric activity (depolarization of the muscle cell membrane [2]) and contributes to the diagnosis of motor disorders [3] and, specifically, that of the most superficial muscles, identifying their contribution (and the importance of the same) in a given task [4]. This technique is based on the detection of the action potential of muscle fibers and motor units in the surrounding tissues or the skin during muscle activity [5]. The signal is represented through voltage, measured in μV. SEMG allows researchers to know the muscle excitation and describe the muscle patterns, giving information about the recruited motor units in a non-invasive way [6].

SEMG is used in a wide variety of disciplines, such as physiology, engineering, biomechanics, medical sciences, and clinical neuroscience [7,8], but in speech therapy, the use of SEMG is not very frequent. Speech–language pathologists and speech therapists use it to help in the evaluation, diagnosis, and therapy of different functions, especially stomatognathic functions such as chewing and swallowing, proper to the orofacial motor area [9], as well as the masticatory muscles' activity [10]. It is a non-invasive technique, easy to apply, and reports muscle activity in real time [11].

The electromyogram obtained is the result of the sum of the motor unit action potentials produced during the contraction of the neuromuscular units [7,12,13]. The amplitude (maximum height of the action potential) is expressed in microvolts, while the frequency is measured in hertz, indicating the number of times the potential is repeated per unit of time (usually in one second) [5].

Recently, high-density surface electromyography [14] has been used to study muscles associated with swallowing. This technique appears to be useful for the analysis of the motor unit recruitment in the suprahyoid muscles—mylohyoid, geniohyoid, digastric, and stylohyoid [15].

The standardization of the recording, analysis, and interpretation of the electromyographic signal is a pending issue and urgently needed, for which interesting projects have been initiated [16].

Research related to the study of the voice together with SEMG is scarce and with a great dispersion in the aspects analyzed, from the sample size to the vocal tasks that have been developed or the muscles studied [3].

The aim of this cross-sectional study is to analyze the most relevant surface electromyographic parameters during vocal emission in Spanish speakers, in a sample of 146 adults (women and men), for the characterization of normality patterns of muscular activity in vocal production tasks.

The hypotheses proposed are as follows: (1) there is a characteristic pattern of SEMG signals associated with normal voice emission, without vocal pathology, and (2) there are differences between sexes.

2. Materials and Methods

2.1. Study Design

Taking into account the objectives of this study, a cross-sectional descriptive design was chosen. Before starting the study, a favorable report on the project was obtained from the Human Research Ethics Committee (CEIH) of Universitat de València with procedure number 1054131.

2.2. Participants

The sample consisted of a total of 146 people (after calculating the sample size), all Spanish speakers, comprising 72 males and 74 females (self-identified as such) between 20 and 50 years of age. All participants who presented a subjective perception of normal voice (both by the person participating in the study and by 3 members of the research team, all voice specialists) were included, as well as those without known vocal pathology (both organic and functional) at the time of the examination and without relevant medical history.

2.3. Materials

The MioTool Face surface electromyograph from Miotec Suite 1.0 (Miotec, Porto Alegre, Brazil) connected to a laptop computer (MSI GP62 2QE Leopard Pro with a Windows 10 operating system) via a USB connection was used to record myoelectric activity. This equipment allows for collecting a maximum of 2000 samples per second.

To capture the electrical potentials (recorded in μV) of the muscles to be studied, the Myotool software incorporated into the electromyograph was used. Of the eight channels that the equipment allows, six were used. The Miograph software (Miotec, Porto Alegre, Brazil) was used for the subsequent visualization and processing of the data.

Adhesive Meditrace Kendall pediatric electrodes—Covidien, Dublin, and Ireland—(Ø = 3 cm) were used, which allowed for more selective recordings due to the spacing between electrodes. These were composed of a white polyethylene foam support with a clasp-shaped adapter and a carbon polymer sensor coated with silver and silver chloride, immersed in a layer of conductive and adhesive hydrogel, to conduct the signal of the muscular electrical activity.

The collection of electromyographic recordings was carried out in a room of the Speech Therapy Clinic of the *Fundació Lluís Alcanyís* of the *Universitat de València*.

2.4. Procedure

During the examination, the subjects who were part of the sample remained seated in a chair with knee and hip flexion of 90°, feet on the floor, back of the hands resting on the legs, and with their gaze fixed on a visual reference to the front. They had support on their backs but not on their heads.

Each participant was asked to swallow to stabilize the larynx, and then the muscles involved in the study were palpated. The neck region corresponding to the suprahyoid, infrahyoid, and sternocleidomastoid muscles was cleaned with gauze soaked in 70° ethyl alcohol (Kern Pharma, Madrid, Spain) before attaching the electrodes. This was intended to decrease the impedance of the skin to better capture the electromyographic signal of the selected muscles and thus provide a better fixation condition for the electrodes [10]. All males who participated in this study had the scanning area completely shaved.

Six electromyography channels (one for each muscle group, namely suprahyoid (SH), infrahyoid (IH), and sternocleidomastoid (ECM), both right (R) and left (L)), and the corresponding 13 disposable electrodes made of hypoallergenic material were used to capture the electrical signal of the muscle: 12 recording electrodes (2 for each channel), separated 1 cm (center to center), and another reference electrode on the olecranon [9]—the most prominent part of the posterior aspect of the elbow—away from the study area to avoid interference.

For the SH muscle group, the electrodes were placed in the submandibular region, longitudinally to the fibers of the mylohyoid and digastric muscles, which are more superficial. For the IH muscle group, they were placed bilaterally and sagittally, 1 cm from the thyroid protuberance. The distance was measured with a digital anthropometric caliper. As for the ECM muscle group, they were positioned in the central part of the muscle in the direction of the clavicle (Figure 1). This is also illustrated anatomically in Figure 2.

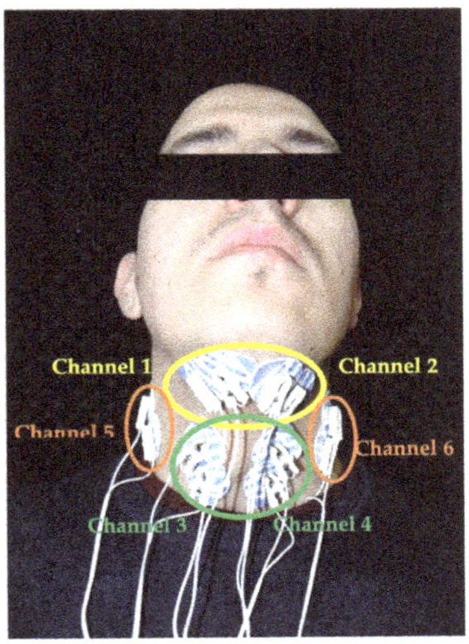

Figure 1. Distribution of SEMG electrodes and channels: Channel 1: R SH; Channel 2: L SH; Channel 3: R IH; Channel 4: L IH; Channel 5: R ECM; Channel 6: L ECM.

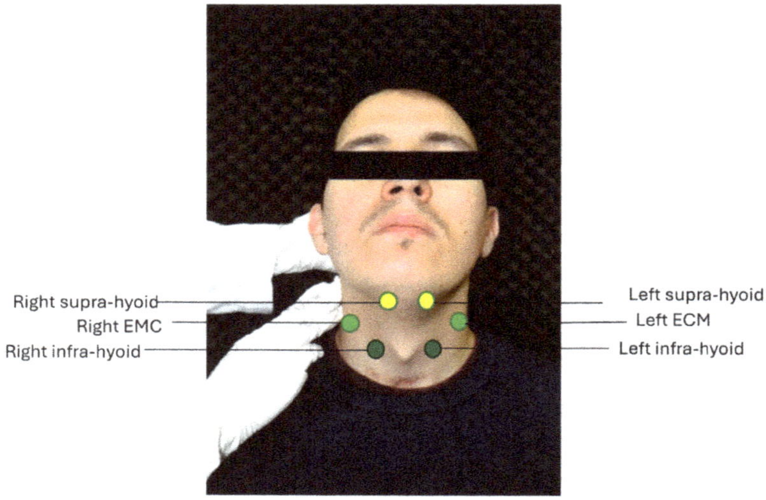

Figure 2. Anatomical positioning of the electrodes.

Surface electromyographic parameters were analyzed in different vocal tasks (Table 1).

Table 1. Surface electromyographic parameters studied in selected vocal tasks.

Vocal Task	Electromyographic Surface Parameters Studied
Reading aloud (SEMG signal normalization task)	Peak (μV)
Vowel /a/ at comfortable frequency and intensity	Mean (μV) Minimum (μV)
Upward *glissando* with the vowel /i/ (low and high part)	Standard deviation (μV)
Rest (time of no vocal activity)	Average frequency (Hz)

Peak (μV): numerical result of the maximum value of electrical activity recorded in the interval analyzed; mean (μV): average value of electrical activity recorded in the interval selected for analysis; minimum (μV): numerical result of the minimum value of electrical activity recorded in the interval analyzed; standard deviation (μV): difference found from the mean value to the extremes of maximum and minimum electrical activity recorded in the interval selected for analysis; mean frequency (Hz) [17].

The selection of the SEMG recording period was carried out in coordination with voice recording. External noise was removed from the SEMG signal with Butterworth-type digital filtering. The following data were then obtained (Table 1): peak (μV) (maximum muscle activity), the mean of muscle activation (μV), the minimum value of muscle activation (μV), and standard deviation (μV) and mean frequency (Hz) of the number of times the action potential is repeated per unit of time.

The dynamic normalization method (with dynamic tasks that were neither isotonic nor isometric) was used in this study, as several authors claim that there is strong evidence of reduced inter-subject variability compared to other normalization methods [13].

The "read-aloud" task was chosen as the baseline activity for signal normalization, as it was felt that it could provide much more information than the other isolated tasks.

Electrical activity was also collected during rest or static assessment [4], which was electrically silent and progressively activated in relation to muscle contraction (Table 1).

2.5. Statistical Analysis

Data were analyzed using SPSS 26.0 (SPSS Inc., Chicago, IL, USA). Cohen's kappa test (κ) was used to determine the concordance between external evaluators, and the Kolmogorov–Smirnov test was used to analyze whether the quantitative variables had a normal distribution. A descriptive analysis was performed for each of the sample variables, namely absolute frequency and percentage for qualitative variables and mean and standard deviation for quantitative variables. The Mann–Whitney U test was used to analyze whether the differences observed were statistically significant when dealing with variables that did not have a normal distribution. To analyze quantitative variables that followed a normal distribution, a *t*-test was applied.

3. Results

During rest (time of no vocal activity), the myoelectric activity (μV) in women was higher than in men for most of the muscles analyzed, while the frequency of the electrical signal (Hz) was higher in men than in women in all the explored muscles. The results obtained in the suprahyoid (C1 and C2) and sternocleidomastoid (C5 and C6) muscles in both sexes showed statistically significant differences (Table 2).

Table 2. Resting muscle electrical activity in men and women.

		Men	Women		Men	Women	
		μV	μV	*p*	Hz	Hz	*p*
C1	Mean	6.67	9.11	<0.01	345.98	311.95	<0.01
	SD	4.27	6.66		59.14	54.79	
C2	Mean	7.50	7.77	<0.05	286.00	266.12	<0.01
	SD	6.08	3.99		41.09	38.81	
C3	Mean	6.05	6.16	0.53	339.03	332.16	0.28
	SD	2.57	2.72		33.18	40.16	
C4	Mean	5.48	5.14	0.90	362.52	358.68	0.19
	SD	3.76	2.39		67.33	37.24	
C5	Mean	12.79	20.40	<0.05	245.20	212.61	<0.01
	SD	10.31	18.41		52.98	54.82	
C6	Mean	6.71	7.03	<0.05	331.22	303.57	<0.01
	SD	6.59	4.49		48.18	51.50	

C1: right suprahyoid channel 1; C2: left suprahyoid channel 2; C3: right infrahyoid channel 3; C4: left infrahyoid channel 4; C5: right ECM channel 5; C6: left ECM channel 6; C7: right ECM channel 6; C8: right ECM channel 6; C9: right ECM channel 6. SD: standard deviation.

Regarding the "comfortable /a/ vowel" task, women obtained higher results than men in most of the analyzed variables and explored muscles, except in the channels referring to the infrahyoid muscles (C3 and C4), where men engaged a greater number of motor units and obtained higher results. Statistically significant differences were observed between men and women (Table 3) both in the mean myoelectric activity (μV) and in the mean frequency (Hz) of the electromyographic parameters in each of the recorded channels, except in Channel 3, referring to the right infrahyoid muscle group ($p = 0.66$). The greatest statistically significant differences were observed in the channels of the suprahyoids (C1 and C2). In the left ECM muscle channel (C6), no differences were observed in terms of mean frequency (Hz), while in the right ECM (C5), they were.

Table 3. Resting muscle electrical activity in the task "vowel /a/ at comfortable frequency and intensity" in men and women.

		Men	Women		Men	Women	
	μV		μV	*p*	Hz	Hz	*p*
C1	Mean	10.11	13.49	<0.01	296.17	275.61	<0.01
	SD	1.86	2.52		41.87	39.16	
C2	Mean	10.56	12.59	<0.01	269.65	253.68	<0.05
	SD	1.94	2.67		38.37	30.69	
C3	Mean	11.91	11.35	0.66	264.13	268.93	0.56
	SD	3.08	2.45		44.51	40.12	
C4	Mean	12.98	10.01	<0.05	265.44	271.87	0.38
	SD	3.56	2.14		4911	38.74	
C5	Mean	12.75	21.47	<0.01	252.79	236.37	<0.01
	SD	1.10	1.59		45.20	57.72	
C6	Mean	8.41	9.99	<0.01	297.31	278.33	0.07
	SD	0.93	1.64		56.99	55.97	

C1: right supra-hyoid channel 1; C2: left supra-hyoid channel 2; C3: right infra-hyoid channel 3; C4: left infra-hyoid channel 4; C5: right ECM channel 5; C6: left ECM channel 6.

There were significant differences in the task "reading aloud" between both sexes (Table 4), in the suprahyoid muscles (C1 and C2) and the peak (μV) and mean (μV) electromyographic parameters ($p < 0.01$).

Table 4. Muscle electrical activity in the task "reading aloud" in men and women.

		Men	Women		Men	Women	
	Mean (μV)		Mean (μV)	*p*	Mean Frequency (Hz)	Mean Frequency (Hz)	*p*
C1	Mean	20.57	29.36	<0.01	229.91	219.99	<0.05
	SD	8.17	10.70		23.03	22.18	
C2	Mean	22.81	29.42	<0.01	219.58	213.80	0.12
	SD	9.72	11.46		19.99	17.43	
C3	Mean	22.72	21.06	0.19	209.85	216.02	0.10
	SD	9.45	7.92		31.18	33.53	
C4	Mean	25.46	18.87	<0.01	202.61	220.49	<0.01
	SD	11.13	7.14		27.51	25.16	
C5	Mean	15.84	21.09	<0.05	237.78	228.84	0.12
	SD	2.84	2.79		30.07	24.47	
C6	Mean	11.15	11.09	0.17	269.53	257.43	0.09
	SD	3.57	2.92		48.32	33.04	

C1: right supra-hyoid channel 1; C2: left supra-hyoid channel 2; C3: right infra-hyoid channel 3; C4: left infra-hyoid channel 4; C5: right ECM channel 5; C6: left ECM channel 6.

In the task "ascending glissando with the vowel /i/", significant differences were observed (Table 5) between men and women in the mean (μV) of the myoelectric activity of the suprahyoid and left infrahyoid and right ECM muscles ($p < 0.01$), as well as the mean electromyographic frequencies (Hz) of the right suprahyoid and left infrahyoid ($p < 0.01$).

In all the previously analyzed tasks, both suprahyoid muscle electrical activity (C1 and C2) and that of the ECM (C5 and C6) were greater ($p < 0.01$) in women, while men presented greater myoelectric activity at the level of infrahyoid muscles (C3 and C4) ($p < 0.01$).

Table 5. Muscle electrical activity in the task "upward glissando with /i/" in men and women.

		Men	Women		Men	Women	
		Mean (μV)	Mean (μV)	p	Mean Frequency (Hz)	Mean Frequency (Hz)	p
C1	Mean	11.34	16.35	<0.01	280.08	254.95	<0.01
	SD	2.04	2.89		41.73	36.54	
C2	Mean	12.80	15.30	<0.01	251.92	239.84	<0.05
	SD	2.50	2.82		36.13	32.66	
C3	Mean	24.34	16.12	<0.01	232.93	249.36	<0.01
	SD	8.34	4.01		46.11	41.77	
C4	Mean	25.92	13.59	<0.01	236.10	263.03	<0.01
	SD	8.60	3.49		47.93	47.69	
C5	Mean	12.88	2096	<0.01	239.73	220.68	<0.01
	SD	1.33	1.33		38.84	42.89	
C6	Mean	7.96	9.37	<0.01	299.98	279.11	<0.01
	SD	0.90	1.41		52.59	41.49	

C1: right supra-hyoid channel 1; C2: left supra-hyoid channel 2; C3: right infra-hyoid channel 3; C4: left infra-hyoid channel 4; C5: right ECM channel 5; C6: left ECM channel 6.

4. Discussion

This study aimed to provide information to establish electromyographic normative parameters, typical of voice tasks and where participants present a euphonic voice, not pathological, to help professionals make clinical decisions. For this purpose, the behavior of the extrinsic musculature of the larynx was assessed at the surface electromyographic level during different vocal tasks in men and women with a normal voice. The methodological procedure was based on the results obtained in a recent systematic review of the scientific literature on normal voice [18]. To the best of our knowledge, no studies have been found in Spanish speakers that analyze normal voice in conjunction with surface electromyography.

Balata (2013) [9] studied the electrical activity of extrinsic laryngeal muscles in people with and without dysphonia. His sample consisted of 36 women and 5 men aged between 28 and 57 years. In his study, he used the same equipment as that used in our work (surface electromyograph, adhesive surface electrodes, and software). His analysis included a smaller number of vocal tasks (vowel /ε/ at comfortable intensity, vowel /ε/ at strong intensity, counting from 20 to 30 at comfortable intensity, and counting from 20 to 30 at strong intensity, together with rest), with three electromyography channels: right and left IH muscles and SH (without specifying the side).

Electromyographic recording depends on electrode placement and application, skin perspiration and temperature, muscle fatigue, contraction speed, muscle bulk, contamination of nearby muscles, subcutaneous fat thickness, or slight variations in the execution of the task [12,13]. Therefore, the signal must be normalized for interpretation and comparison, which is not simple [2]. Lehman and McGill (1999) [12] proposed that electromyographic normalization be performed by means of a reference task, through which the activity values of the electrical signal are expressed as a percentage of the electrical activity of the muscles to be studied during contraction.

The aim is to have a standardized and reliable reference value, by changing the data scale from microvolts to percentages to compare the electrical activity of muscles in a task over time between different muscles and participants [19–21].

Research dedicated to the study of the voice in conjunction with SEMG is limited and studies different variables and uses different methodological components such as the muscle groups analyzed, the phonatory tasks recorded, materials, sample size, etc., making it difficult to compare results.

Although SENIAM (surface electromyography for the non-invasive assessment of muscles) is recommended in Europe for the correct placement and location of sensors and is used as the methodology for signal processing, there is currently no specific protocol on the placement of sensors in the extrinsic muscles of the larynx (specifically the suprahyoid

(SH) and infrahyoid (IH)) and neck (part of which is the sternocleidomastoid (ECM)). In our case, we decided to place them as previously explained and as shown in Figure 1. Obviously, a consensus standard would be desirable to unify the methodology in this type of research.

In the present study, we chose to study the ECM muscles bilaterally (in addition to the SH and IH) since, according to Behlau and Pontes (1995) [22], these muscles tend to elevate the rib cage constantly, along with the laryngeal elevation and restriction of movements in subjects with vocal pathology. Authors such as Ramos et al. (2018) [23] state that ECMs are muscles in which people with vocal pathology tend to present more pain.

There are other studies using SEMG with vocally normal and dysphonic subjects, although with different objectives. The study by Silvério (1999) [24] analyzed the electrical activity of the ECM and trapezius muscles (upper fibers) in normal and dysphonic individuals. Sapir et al. (2000) [25] evaluated variations in the fundamental frequency together with electrical activity but, in this case, induced by mechanical disturbance of the larynx. Silvério (2002) [26] studied vocal evaluation together with the electrical activity of SH and ECM muscles but in women aged between 20 and 40 years with temporomandibular dysfunction, at rest and phonation. Once again, the variability of the published studies makes comparative analysis difficult.

The recording of the SEMG data required, initially, the precise selection of the period to be studied, taking the time of the voice recordings as a reference. In this way, the exact time window was calculated with SEMG, since it only uses the time variable as a guide for the analysis. To perform both recordings at the same time, the "start" option was selected simultaneously, but on some occasions, the SEMG recording took a few milliseconds longer to start than the vocal recording. For this reason, it was decided to count from the end, stopping the recording again at the same time and ensuring accuracy in data extraction.

The applied digital filtering, Butterworth type [9], attenuates the undesirable frequencies of the signal through two second-order filters, a high-pass filter at 20 Hz that lets through the frequencies above that frequency and a low-pass filter at 450 Hz, letting through the frequencies below that frequency [27], which were configured as cutoff frequencies to define the upper and lower filtering limits since the highest-frequency components contained in the SEMG signals are below 400–500 Hz [7].

The dynamic normalization method (with dynamic tasks that were neither isotonic nor isometric) was used in this study, as it has been revealed that there is strong evidence of reduced inter-subject variability compared to other normalization methods [13,20]. The "read-aloud" task was chosen as the reference activity for signal normalization, as it was considered to be one that could provide more information than the other isolated tasks. Electrical activity during rest (statically) was also recorded, which is electrically silent and allows for the assessment of the muscle without load [28]. In a general way, it can be seen how "reading aloud" is the task that recruits more motor units than the others, taking "rest" or "no muscle activity" as a reference.

During the task "upward glissando with the vowel /i/", the mean myoelectric activity was slightly higher in the infrahyoid and ECM muscles at low frequencies, while the mean myoelectric activity of the suprahyoids was slightly higher at high frequencies. A plausible explanation for the higher amplitude of the ECM electrical signal at low frequencies may be due to the onset of inhalation (high/clavicular breathing may have occurred at most phonatory onsets) or a very rapid inhalation at the time of first uttering a low frequency [29]. Another reasonable, although unconfirmed, explanation would be the possible involvement of ECMs in an attempt to lower the larynx at lower pitches. The higher amplitude at high frequencies in the supra-hyoid muscles is due to the laryngeal rise that occurs during higher-pitched vocal emissions, due to the increased activity of the cricothyroid muscle responsible for the progressive elevation of the vocal ligament [30,31].

In our work, in general (since several SEMG channels were analyzed in different vocal tasks), women presented a higher mean myoelectric activity (μV) at the SH and ECM muscle levels than men, while the mean frequency of the electrical signal (Hz) was higher in men than in women. This may be due to the fact that the higher the amplitude of the SEMG (μV) (i.e., the higher the recruitment of motor units), the lower the conduction velocity of muscle action potentials (i.e., the lower the SEMG frequencies (Hz)) [32]. The changes that may occur at the level of the amplitude and frequency of the SEMG signal are related to constant changes in the performance of force, the length of the muscle fibers, the placement/position of the surface electrodes, and the active muscle fibers during the different tasks [33].

An important aspect to take into account is the variety of vocal tasks that were studied in the present study. It is important to consider that continuous speech is a much more complex task than sustained vocal emission because, in the former, many more orofacial structures are activated.

The results obtained regarding the mean muscle electrical activity of the SH and ECM muscles, both in men and women, presented statistically significant differences in our work, aspects that cannot be compared due to the lack of similar studies. Research by Silvério (1999) [24] and Balata (2013) [9] compared dysphonic and euphonic subjects and did not analyze differences between sexes. The analysis of SEMG results revealed a large interindividual variation, even in subjects performing the same task [34,35].

The results of the present study, performed on a population without pathology, show differences by gender, but these obviously cannot be extrapolated to populations with dysphonia. On the other hand, the scarcity of evidence in this field does not allow us to do so either.

SEMG is not widely used in clinical speech therapy practice (recognition of dysfunctions) or the control of therapy; these cases involve procedures for recording information that is not uniform, which implies the translation of the analyses performed [4]. It is evident that without a methodological standardization that minimizes individual variations [24], it is not possible to adequately broaden the spectrum of knowledge in this field, since the capacity for comparison with other studies is limited.

5. Conclusions

Within the characteristics and limitations of this study, the following conclusions can be drawn:

SEMG provides valid and objective data on the extrinsic muscular activity of the larynx during phonation, but this tool cannot precisely define such markers since the electrophysiological assessment of phonation is subject to many individual variables. On the other hand, we wish to highlight the potential of surface electromyography as biofeedback and the benefits that its use can bring from a clinical point of view.

The dynamic tasks related to connected speech best describe the myoelectric behavior of the extrinsic structures of the larynx involved in the phonatory process. The mean myoelectric activity of the suprahyoid musculature and that of the sternocleidomastoid muscles was higher in women, whereas the mean myoelectric activity of the infrahyoid musculature was higher in men.

Therefore, the proposed hypotheses are accepted. The behavior of the SEMG signals was analyzed, and differences between sexes were observed for the studied population. However, it is necessary to establish a system of standardization of the scans and conduct further research to make the data comparable with each other and with other populations.

Author Contributions: Conceptualization, C.P.-H. and V.R.-C.; methodology, C.P.-H.; software, C.P.-H. and J.L.S.; validation, V.R.-C., L.B.-L. and L.F.; formal analysis, V.R.-C. and L.F.; investigation, C.P.-H.; resources, L.F. and J.L.S.; data curation, C.P.-H. and V.R.-C.; writing—original draft preparation, C.P.-H.; writing—review and editing, C.P.-H., L.F. and J.L.S.; visualization, V.R.-C., L.B.-L. and L.F.; supervision, V.R.-C. and L.B.-L.; project administration, V.R.-C.; funding acquisition, L.F. All authors have read and agreed to the published version of the manuscript.

Funding: This research received no external funding.

Institutional Review Board Statement: This study was conducted in accordance with the Declaration of Helsinki and approved by the Human Research Ethics Committee (CEIH) of Universitat de València (procedure number 1054131).

Informed Consent Statement: Informed consent was obtained from all subjects involved in the study. Consent was obtained prior to the inclusion of the patient's photographs.

Data Availability Statement: Not applied.

Conflicts of Interest: The authors declare no conflicts of interest.

References

1. Valentino, W.L.; Park, J.; Alnouri, G.; Gracely, E.J.; Tami, A.; Vance, D.; Palmer, J.; Sataloff, R.T. Diagnostic Value of Acoustic a Aerodynamic Measurements in Vocal Fold Movement Disorders and their Correlation with Laryngeal Electromyography a Voice Handicap Index. *J. Voice* **2021**, *35*, 497.e1–497.e4. [CrossRef] [PubMed]
2. Wang, F.; Yiu, E.M. Predicting Dysphonia by Measuring Surface Electromyographic Activity of the Supralaryngeal Muscle *Speech Lang. Hear. Res.* **2024**, *67*, 740–752. [CrossRef] [PubMed]
3. Balata, P.M.M.M.; da Silva, H.J.; Rocha de Moraes, K.J.; Pernambuco, L.A.; de Moraes, S.R.A. Use of Surface electromyograph phonation studies: An integrative review. *Int. Arch. Otorhinolaryngol.* **2013**, *17*, 329–339. [CrossRef] [PubMed]
4. Estrada Muñoz, C.A. Surface electromyography as a method for the study of anaerobic aerobic transition. *Ergon. Res. Dev.* 2 1, 63–80. Available online: http://revistasacademicas.udec.cl/index.php/Ergonomia_Investigacion/article/view/1279 (acces on 10 January 2024).
5. Wang, F.; Yiu, E.M. Surface electromyographic (sEMG) activity of the suprahyoid and sternocleidomastoid muscles in pitch a loudness control. *Front. Physiol.* **2023**, *14*, 1147795. [CrossRef] [PubMed]
6. Shabani, Q.; ShaterzadehYazdi, M.J.; Soltani, M.; Behdarvandan, A.; Najarzadeh, Z.; Naderifar, E.; Dastoorpour, M.; Moradi, Rahimifar, P. The effects of transcutaneous electrical nerve stimulation on muscle activity pattern in professional voice users w muscle tension dysphonia using surface electromyography data: A pilot study. *Am. J. Otolaryngol.* **2023**, *44*, 103911. [CrossRef] [PubMed]
7. McManus, L.; Lowery, M.; Merletti, R.; Søgaard, K.; Besomi, M.; Clancy, E.A.; van Dieën, J.H.; Hug, F.; Wrigley, T.; Besier, T.; e Consensus for Experimental Design in Electromyography (CEDE) project: Terminology matrix. *J. Electromyogr. Kinesiol.* **2021**, 102565. [CrossRef]
8. Di Nardo, F.; Fioretti, S. Accuracy of EMG linear envelope in identifying the peak of muscular activity during walking. *G Posture* **2024**, *111*, 185–190. [CrossRef] [PubMed]
9. Balata, P.M.M. Atividade Elétrica dos Músculos Extrínsecos da Laringe em Sujeitos com e sem Disfonía. Master's The Universidade Federal de Pernambuco, Recife, Brazil, 2013. ATTENA-Repositório Digital da UFPE. Available online: ht //repositorio.ufpe.br/handle/123456789/12592 (accessed on 4 March 2024).
10. Wang, X.; Liu, H.; Zhang, X.; Qu, Z.; Zhao, J. Effect of transcutaneous electrical nerve stimulation (TENS) on the electromyograp activity of human masticatory muscles in young people with normal occlusion. *J. Prosthet. Dent.* 2024, *in press*. [CrossRef]
11. Rosell-Clari, V. Orofacial alterations and surface electromyography in neurodevelopmental disorders. *Rev. Neurol.* **2017**, (Suppl. S1), S85–S88.
12. Lehman, G.J.; McGill, S.M. The importance of normalization in the interpretation of surface electromyography: A proo principle. *J. Manip. Physiol. Ther.* **1999**, *22*, 444–446. [CrossRef] [PubMed]
13. Vojtech, J.M.; Mitchell, C.L.; Raiff, L.; Kline, J.C.; De Luca, G. Prediction of Voice Fundamental Frequency and Intensity fr Surface Electromyographic Signals of the Face and Neck. *Vibration* **2022**, *5*, 692–710. [CrossRef] [PubMed]
14. Merletti, R.; Holobar, A.; Farina, D. Analysis of motor units with high-density surface electromyography. *J. Electromyogr. Kine* **2008**, *18*, 879–890. [CrossRef] [PubMed]
15. Yoshikawa, K.; Nakamori, M.; Ushio, K.; Toko, M.; Yamada, H.; Nishikawa, Y.; Fukuoka, T.; Maruyama, H.; Mikami, Y.J. Analy of the suprahyoid muscles during tongue elevation: High-density surface electromyography as a novel tool for swallowing-rela muscle assessment. *Oral Rehabil.* 2024, *Online ahead of print*. [CrossRef] [PubMed]
16. Hodges, P.W. Consensus for experimental design in electromyography, project. *J. Electromyogr. Kinesiol.* **2020**, *50*, 102 [CrossRef]
17. Da Silva, H.J. *Protocolos de Eletromiografia de Superfície em Fonoaudiología*; Pró-Fono: São Paulo, Brasil, 2013.
18. Puig-Herreros, C.; Sanz, J.L.; Barona, L.; Rosell-Clari, V. Acoustic, myoelectric, and aerodynamic parameters of euphonic a dysphonic voices: A systematic review of clinical studies. *Appl. Sci.* **2021**, *11*, 8191. [CrossRef]
19. De Luca, C.J. The use of surface electromyography in biomechanics. *J. Appl. Biomech.* **1997**, *13*, 135–163. [CrossRef]
20. Burden, A.; Bartlett, R. Normalization of EMG amplitude: An evaluation and comparison of old and new methods. *Med. E Phys.* **1999**, *21*, 247–257. [CrossRef] [PubMed]
21. Ball, N.; Scurr, J. An assessment of the reliability and standardization of tests used to elicit reference muscular actions electromyographical normalization. *J. Electromyogr. Kinesiol.* **2010**, *20*, 81–88. [CrossRef]
22. Behlau, M.; Pontes, P. *Avaliação e Tratamento das Disfonías*; Lovise: São Paulo, Brasil, 1995.

Ramos, A.C.; Floro, R.L.; Ribeiro, V.V.; Brasolotto, A.G.; Silvério, K.C.A. Musculoskeletal pain and vcice-related quality of life in dysphonic and non-dysphonic subjects. *J. Voice* **2018**, *32*, 307–313. [CrossRef]
Silvério, K.C.A. Atividade Elétrica dos Músculos Esternocleidomastoideo e Trapézio: Fibras Superiores em Individuos Normais e Disfônicos. Master's Thesis, Universidade Estadual de Campinas, São Paulo, Brasil, 1999. Repositório da Produção Científica e Intelectual da Unicamp. Available online: https://repositorio.unicamp.br/acervo/detalhe/175714 (accessed on 4 March 2024).
Sapir, S.; Baker, K.K.; Larson, C.R.; Ramig, L.O. Short-latency changes in voice F0 and neck surface EMG induced by mechanical perturbations of the larynx during sustained vowel phonation. *J. Speech Lang. Hear. Res.* **2000**, *43*, 268–276. [CrossRef] [PubMed]
Silvério, K.C.A. Avaliação Vocal e Atividade Eletrica dos Musculos Supra-Hioideos e Esternocleidomastoideo em Individuos com Desordem Temporomandibular Miogenica em Situações de Repouso e Fonação. Doctoral Thesis, Universidade Estadual de Campinas, São Paulo, Brasil, 2002. Repositório da Produção Científica e Intelectual da Unicamp. [CrossRef]
De Sá Ferreira, A.; Silva Guimarães, F.; Silva, J.G. Aspectos metodológicos da eletromiografia de superfície: Considerações sobre os sinais e processamentos para estudo da função neuromuscular. *Rev. Bras. Ciências Esporte* **2010**, *31*, 11–30. Available online: https://www.redalyc.org/articulo.oa?id=401338541002 (accessed on 4 March 2024).
Estrada, C.A. Electromiografía de superficie como método para el estudio de la transición aeróbica anaeróbica. *Ergon. Investig. Y Desarro.* **2019**, *1*, 63–80.
Pettersen, V.; Westgaard, R.H. The activity patterns of neck muscles in professional classical singing. *J. Voice* **2005**, *19*, 238–251. [CrossRef] [PubMed]
Giovanni, A.; Lagier, A.; Henrich, N. Fisiología de la fonació. *EMC-Otorrinolaringol.* **2014**, *43*, 1–16. [CrossRef]
Marmouset, F.; Hammoudi, K.; Bobillier, C.; Morinière, S. Fisiología de la deglución normal. *EMC-Otorrinolaringol.* **2015**, *44*, 1–12. [CrossRef]
Crozara, L.F.; Castro, A.; De Almeida Neto, A.F.; Laroche, D.P.; Cardozo, A.C.; Gonçalves, M. Utility of electromyographic fatigue threshold during treadmill running. *Muscle Nerve* **2015**, *52*, 1030–1039. [CrossRef]
Bonato, P. Recent advancements in the analysis of dynamic EMG data. *IEEE Eng. Med. Biol. Mag. Q. Mag. Eng. Med. Biol. Soc.* **2001**, *20*, 29–32. [CrossRef] [PubMed]
Balogh, I.; Hansson, G.A.; Ohlsson, K.; Strömberg, U.; Skerfving, S. Interindividual variation of physical load in a work task. *Scand. J. Work. Environ. Health* **1999**, *25*, 57–66. [CrossRef]
Yiu, E.M.; Lau, G.W.H.; Wang, F. Fatigue-Related Change in Surface Electromyographic Activities of the Perilaryngeal Muscles. *J. Speech Lang. Hear. Res.* **2023**, *66*, 98–109. [CrossRef]

Journal of
Personalized Medicine

MDPI

Systematic Review

Efficacy of Internet-Based Therapies for Tinnitus: A Systemati Review and Meta-Analysis of Randomized Controlled Trials

Egidio Sia [1], Giancarlo Tirelli [1], Annalisa Gatto [1], Chiara Angela Mineo [1], Kaveri Curlin [2] and Mehdi Abouzari [2]

[1] Department of Medical, Surgical and Health Sciences, Section of Otolaryngology, University of Trieste, 34149 Trieste, Italy
[2] Division of Neurotology and Skull Base Surgery, Department of Otolaryngology-Head and Neck Surgery, University of California, Irvine, CA 92697, USA
* Correspondence: mabouzar@hs.uci.edu; Tel.: +1-714-509-6096

Abstract: Background: Tinnitus presents a major public health challenge, impacting quality of life. With conventional therapies being often time-consuming and costly, interest in Internet-based treatments, such as auditory treatments and Internet-based cognitive behavioral therapy, has grown due to their improved patient adherence. This meta-analysis aims to review existing scientific literature to assess the effectiveness of Internet-based therapies (IBTs) in treating tinnitus. Methods: Studies up to February 2024 using the Tinnitus Functional Index (TFI), Tinnitus Handicap Inventory (THI), or Tinnitus Reactions Questionnaire (TRQ) to monitor tinnitus before and after IBTs were searched in PubMed, Google Scholar, Web of Science, and the Cochrane Central Register of Controlled Trials. Variation of the score with time was analyzed and a comparison was made with non-IBT studies. Treatment effects were analyzed using Cohen's d model. Results: A total of 14 articles were considered, with a total of 1574 patients. Significant improvements in questionnaire scores were noted post-treatment. In the IBT group, THI and TFI decreased by 17.97 and 24.56 points, respectively (Cohen's d THI: 0.85; TFI: 0.80). In the control group, THI and TFI decreased by 13.7 and 4.25 points, respectively (Cohen's d THI: 0.55; TFI: 0.10). Conclusions: Internet-based therapies showed reliable effectiveness, possibly due to improved patient compliance, accessibility, cost-effectiveness, and customization.

Keywords: tinnitus; internet-based treatment; Tinnitus Functional Index (TFI); Tinnitus Handicap Inventory (THI); Tinnitus Reactions Questionnaire (TRQ)

1. Introduction

Tinnitus, colloquially referred to as "ringing in the ears", is "an auditory sensation without an external sound stimulation or meaning, which can be lived as an unpleasant experience, possibly impacting quality of life" [1]. Over the past 20–30 years, it has emerged as a serious public health issue, affecting 760 million people worldwide [2,3]. Tinnitus is a symptom, not a disease, and although it is often associated with curable and non-critical conditions, it impacts quality of life, partly due to inherent challenges in its treatment [4]. In fact, it often manifests without any objective signs, and due to inadequate understanding of its pathology, it can be a symptom of various disorders such as otological, orofacial, cardiovascular, and neurological diseases [5]. Tinnitus may originate from cochlear abnormalities or hearing loss and is then maintained by neural changes in the central auditory system, with altered neuronal activity [5]. Arterial and arteriovenous pulsatile tinnitus could result from arterial stenosis, skull base anatomical variants, or vascular skull base tumors, while somatic inputs such as temporomandibular disorders can influence tinnitus perception in a condition known as "somatosensory tinnitus" [6,7]. As a neurological disorder, it is known that tinnitus may be associated with migraine phenomena, as both are similarly elusive in etiology but possibly share a pathophysiology linked by the central nervous system [8]. The absence of an objective measure for tinnitus has resulted in self-report questionnaires being the preferred method to evaluate tinnitus symptoms and quantify the degree to which quality of life is affected negatively [9]. There are several tinnitus questionnaires available, with widely used ones including the Tinnitus Reaction Questionnaire (TRQ) [10], Tinnitus Handicap Inventory (THI) [11], and Tinnitus Functional Index (TFI) [12]. The THI is a 25-item survey with three subscales: functional (12 items), emotional (eight items), and catastrophic response (five items), and is a robust measure of tinnitus impact on everyday life. The TFI, also a 25-item index, scales tinnitus severity, identifies domains affecting it and measures treatment-related changes, with scores ranging from 0 to 100, categorized into five severity levels from 'not a problem' to 'very big problem'. The TRQ consists of 26 items rated from 0 to 4, summed into a total score from 0 to 104, and describes the distress associated with tinnitus. In all three questionnaires, higher scores correspond to greater severity of tinnitus. After assessing the severity of tinnitus and its impact on quality of life, treatment in these patients should focus on addressing the underlying or concurrent disorder (if present) and implementing specific treatments aimed at reducing the severity of the tinnitus. Treatments for managing tinnitus include psychological interventions such as counseling and psychoeducation, auditory stimulation such as sound therapy, and, when necessary, interventions to reduce distress such as relaxation therapy [2,13,14]. Based on the possibility that tinnitus is linked to high spontaneous neuronal activity, brain stimulation therapies, such as transcranial magnetic stimulation, transcranial direct current stimulation, and deep brain stimulation, represent valid treatment options for these patients [5,15–17]. Furthermore, in recent years, there has been a growing interest in Internet-based therapies (IBTs). These approaches hold promise in overcoming some of the limitations associated with conventional therapies, ensuring accessibility, cost reduction, and consequently enhancing patient compliance. They include questionnaires, auditory treatments, internet-based cognitive behavioral therapy (iCBT), and games present in different operating systems for tinnitus monitoring and management [4].

The purpose of this study was to review peer-reviewed publications on the effectiveness of internet-based therapies for tinnitus to analyze the efficacy of these treatments. The primary aim was to assess tinnitus improvement resulting from IBT by examining how patient questionnaire scores (THI, TFI, and TRQ) varied over time, reported as medians and with a 95% confidence interval. The secondary objective was to compare outcomes between patients receiving IBT (case group) and non-IBT patients (control group treatment, CGT). This meta-analysis intentionally selected studies concerning IBTs that vary significantly from one another, both in terms of delivery methods (e.g., smartphone-based, web-based, computer-based) and types of therapy (e.g., cognitive-behavioral therapy, music therapy). This approach has allowed us to include a larger number of studies and to analyze the overall effectiveness of IBT compared to face-to-face therapies.

2. Materials and Methods

2.1. Search Strategy

This manuscript is based on the PRISMA guidelines. PROSPERO registration was completed (ID 565308). The databases PubMed, Google Scholar, Web of Science, and the Cochrane Central Register of Controlled Trials were searched up to February 2024. The bibliographic research was conducted by a health sciences librarian. The search syntax was adapted for each database to account for variation in thesaurus terms/controlled vocabulary across databases. Keywords were used to identify paper sources that included the following: (1) the condition being studied ("tinnitus"); (2) the proposed intervention ("therapy" OR "intervention" OR "treatment"); (3) the method of intervention delivery ("mobile" OR "internet" OR "in-person"). Covidence software (https://www.covidence.org/ accessed on 1 July 2024) was used for the research and to deduplicate results. Exact search terms used in each database are presented in Appendix A.

2.2. Study Selection

Only studies that quantified the intensity of tinnitus using the TFI, THI, and TRQ were considered. Only full text articles were included. The PICO framework was employed to clearly define study eligibility, as follows: (P) patients with tinnitus; (I) Internet-based therapies (including mobile, internet, and in-person); (C) control patients; (O) variation of tinnitus intensity based on the chosen questionnaires.

The exclusion criteria were as follows: (1) reviews, editorials, and non-full-text articles; (2) non-English language studies; (3) studies that evaluated a therapeutic period shorter than 6 weeks; (4) studies containing aggregated and non-extractable data, or duplicated data from previously published work.

2.3. Data Extraction

An electronic data-collection form was used to collect the data. The following information were collected: (1) study information: author, year of publication, country of the cohort, type of study; (2) Internet-based therapies: modality, type of treatment, duration of treatment, type of questionnaire, number of patients pre- and post-treatment, pre- and post-treatment median and standard deviation across various questionnaires; (3) follow-up: number of patients, median and standard deviation across various questionnaires at 2, 3, 6, and 12 months; (4) control group: treatment type, number of patients, median and standard deviation across different questionnaires before and after treatment.

2.4. Statistical Analysis

The median scores across different questionnaires, along with the number of patients and standard deviations for both cases and controls, were extracted from the studies. A 95% confidence interval (CI) was calculated for each questionnaire, assessing scores pre-treatment and at the end of treatment. Additionally, scores harvested 12 months after the beginning of therapy were considered in the cases group. Calculations were performed using random effects models by DerSimonian and Laird, employing a weighted average approach that assigned each study a weight proportional to its precision and incorporated both within- and between-study variability [18]. The results of the meta-analysis were graphically presented using forest plots, which included summary estimates and a corresponding 95% CI. Differences in the effect size among the cases over time and disparities in outcomes between cases and controls were assessed using Cohen's d model. All statistical analysis were calculated using RStudio Desktop, version 2023.09.0+463.

3. Results

3.1. Search Results and Study Selection

Once the duplicates were eliminated, 259 items were screened, leading to the exclusion of 156 articles based on the title. The full text of the remaining 103 articles was further reviewed, and 15 articles met the inclusion criteria for the meta-analysis, as depicted in Figure 1. Data describing the characteristics of the included studies are reported in the Table presented in Appendix B.

The work of Searchfield and colleagues [19] was excluded from the statistical analysis due to the presentation of its results, which were not compatible with our data collection and statistical analysis procedures. The included articles [20–33] involved 1574 patients. Among the selected articles, nine studies were randomized control trials (RCTs), two were pilot trials, one was a repeated measure design, one an effectiveness trial, one a preliminary study, and one a single group open trial. Two of the articles [23,28] described RCTs where patients were monitored using two questionnaires; for this reason, they were considered separately for our statistical analysis. Two other studies [25,26] were three-arm RCTs, with, respectively, two case groups and two control groups. For this reason, they were considered as different studies for our statistical analysis; thus, they were counted as four separated studies.

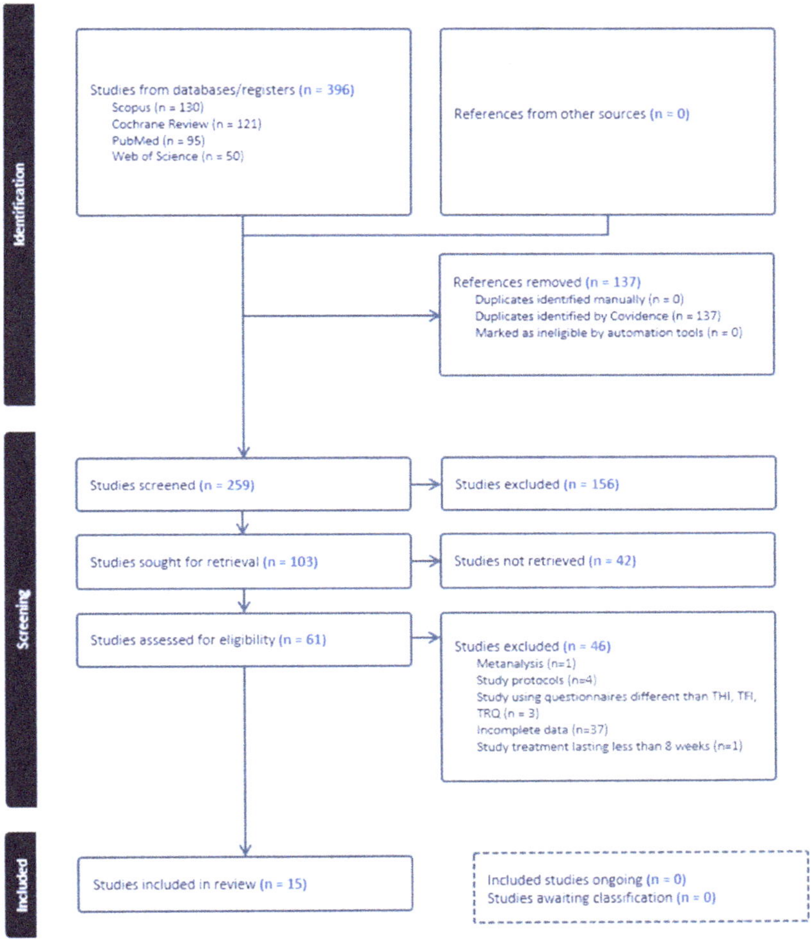

Figure 1. Selection of articles according to the PRISMA statement flow diagram.

3.2. Pre- and Post-Internet-Based Treatment (IBT) Differences

A total of 987 patients underwent IBT between 8 and 12 weeks. In particular, 800 participants underwent iCBT treatment (internet-delivered cognitive behavioral therapy) [21–28,31], 93 iCBT with therapist guidance [30,32], 26 were subjected to music therapy [29], 35 participated in iACT (internet-delivered acceptance and commitment therapy) [25], 20 engaged in a combined treatment approach of iCBT and music therapy [20], and 61 underwent virtual reality treatment [33]. In terms of outcomes, before commencing the treatment, 405 patients were assessed with the THI questionnaire, 383 with the TFI questionnaire, and 319 with the TRQ. At the conclusion of the treatment, a total of 812 patients had their tinnitus assessed, with 355, 297, and 209 patients, respectively, using the THI, TFI, and TRQ questionnaires. According to the random effects model calculation (Figure 2), the mean THI score in patients who underwent Internet-based therapy was 48.64 (95% CI: 38.18–59.11) at pre-treatment, decreased to 30.67 (95% CI: 19.87–41.46) at post-treatment, and slightly increased to 36.44 (95% CI: 15.34–57.53) at the 1-year follow-up. Data regarding TFI score are presented in Figure 3: at pre-treatment, the TFI score was 57.02 (95% CI: 40.93–73.11), which decreased to 32.43 (95% CI: 13.49–51.38) at post-treatment and remained relatively stable at the 1-year follow-up [33.43 (95% CI: −0.77–67.62)]. Finally, the mean TRQ score (Figure 4) at pre-treatment was 29.62 (95% CI: 5.79–53.45), and at post-treatment, it was 20.66 (95% CI: −2.70–44.02). Data on tinnitus status at the 1-year follow-up, assessed using THI and TFI questionnaires, are provided in Appendix C.

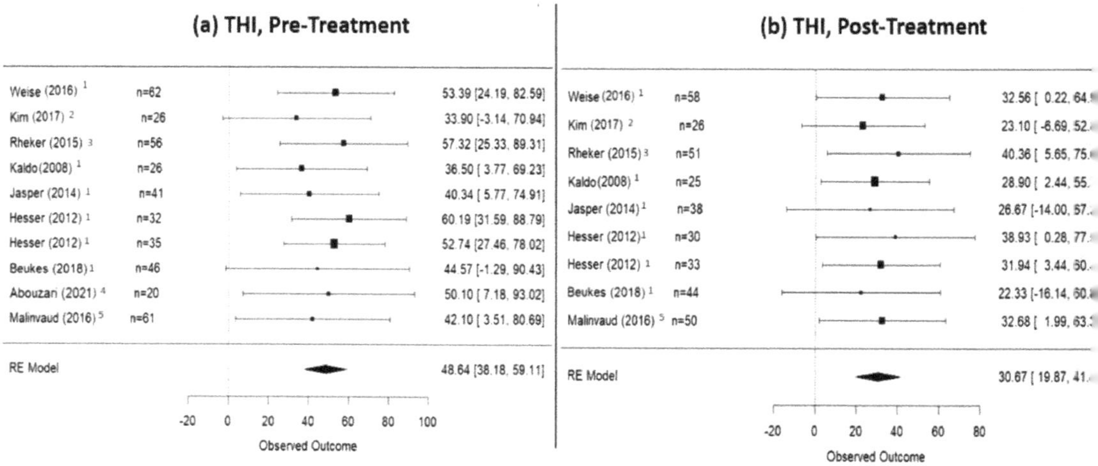

Figure 2. THI scores in patients who underwent internet-based therapies. (**a**) Pre-treatment scores; (**b**) post-treatment scores. This figure shows a THI decrease of 17.97 points (from 48.64 pre-treatment to 30.67 post-treatment). 1: iCBT studies; 2: a sound therapy study; 3: an iCBT + therapist study; 4: an iCBT + sound therapy study; 5: a virtual reality study [21,23,26,27,29–32,34].

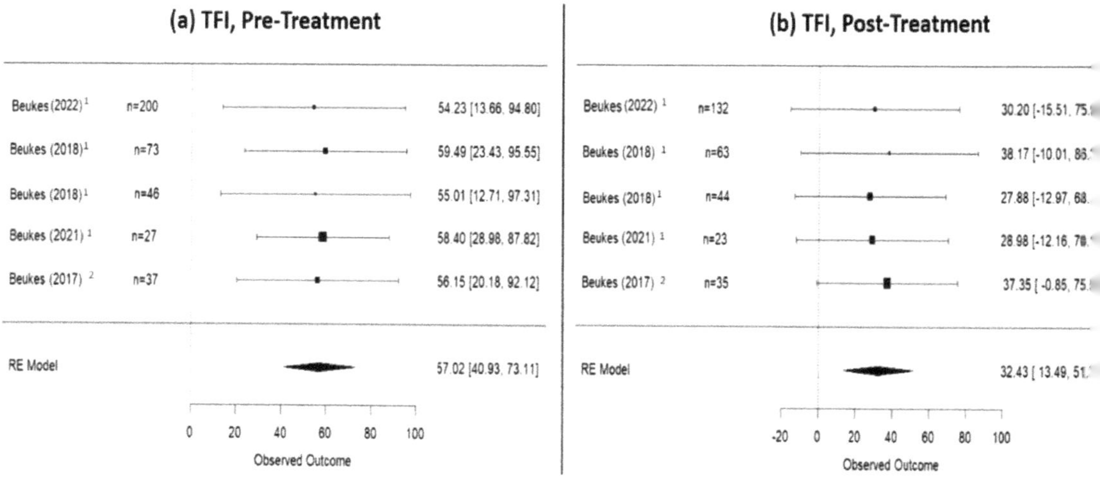

Figure 3. TFI scores in patients who underwent internet-based therapies. (**a**) Pre-treatment scores; (**b**) post-treatment scores. This figure shows a TFI decrease of 24.59 points (from 57.02 pre-treatment to 32.43 post-treatment). 1: iCBT studies; 2: an iCBT + therapist study [22–25,33].

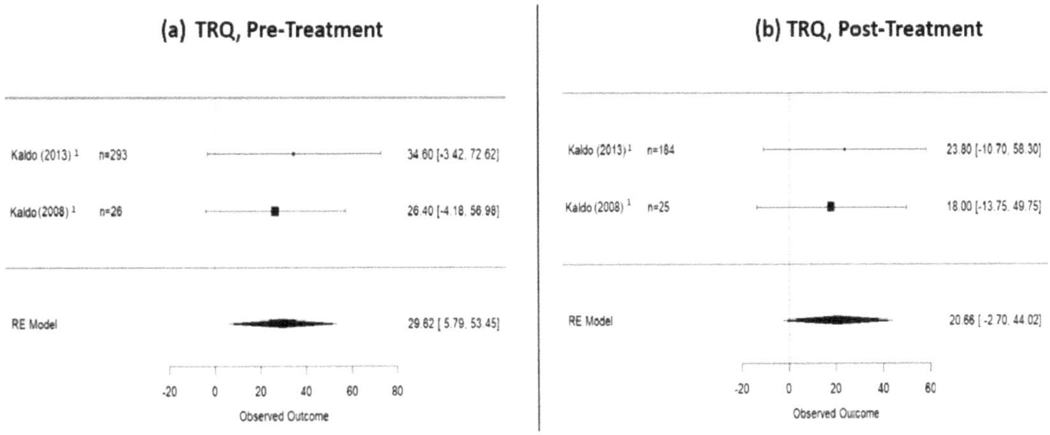

Figure 4. TRQ scores in patients who underwent internet-based therapies. (**a**) Pre-treatment scores; (**b**) post-treatment scores. This figure shows a TRQ decrease of 8.96 points (from 29.62 pre-treatment to 20.66 post-treatment). 1: iCBT studies [28,29].

3.3. Control Group Treatment (CGT)

The total number of patients included in the CGT was 494. Specifically, 221 patients participated in a discussion forum (DF), 179 underwent cognitive-behavioral therapy (CBT), 46 received face-to-face therapy (F2F), and 48 underwent music therapy. Before commencing the treatment, 373 patients were assessed using THI, 119 using TFI, and 25 using TRQ. At the conclusion of treatment, the total number of controls was 414, with 332, 116, and 24 using THI, TFI, and TRQ, respectively, to assess tinnitus improvement. According to the random effects model calculation, the mean THI score in the control group was 51.88 (95% CI: 40.00–63.77) at pre-treatment, notably decreasing to 38.16 (95% CI: 25.25–51.80) at post-treatment. The mean TFI score at pre-treatment was 57.99 (95% CI: 30.61–85.37), decreasing to 53.74 (95% CI: 46.19–61.29) at post-treatment. Due to having only one study with TRQ scores in the control group, a forest plot for TRQ values in the control group was not created [28]. Data are shown in Figure 5.

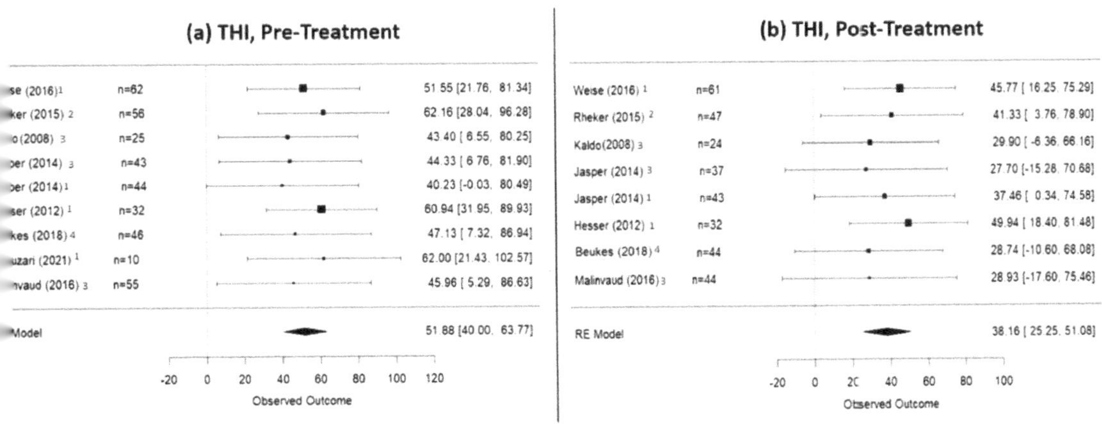

Figure 5. *Cont.*

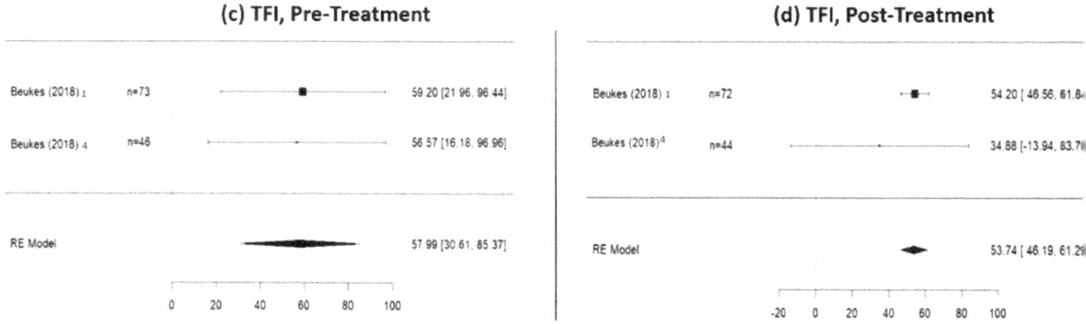

Figure 5. THI and TFI scores of the control group treatment (CGT, patients who did not undergo internet-based therapies). This figure shows a THI decrease of 13.72 points and a TFI decrease of 4.25 in the CGT group. (**a**) Pre-treatment THI scores; (**b**) post-treatment THI scores; (**c**) pre-treatment TFI scores; (**d**) post-treatment TFI scores. 1: studies with DF as control group treatment; 2: a study with iCBT as control group treatment; 3: studies with CBT as control group treatment; 4: a study with F2F as control group treatment [21,23,24,26,27,29,31,32,34].

3.4. Size Effect Analysis

In order to measure the effect size of IBT, calculations were made according to a Cohen's d model to highlight the standardized difference between the means of two groups. Cohen's d values should be interpreted as follows: small effect (around 0.2), medium effect (around 0.5), and large effect (around 0.8 or higher). Cohen's d was calculated based on the pre- vs. post-IBT variation in the scores of THI and TFI, aiming to highlight the effect of IBT on tinnitus (Table 1). The Cohen's d for THI and TFI was 0.85 and 0.71, respectively, indicating a high effect of the treatment on THI and a moderate–high effect on TFI. Cohen's d for TRQ variation was 0.19, indicating a low effect of IBT.

Table 1. Cohen's d calculation among different groups.

Groups Compared	Questionnaire Used	Cohen's d Calculation
Pre- vs. post-IBT	THI	0.8460
Pre- vs. post-IBT	TFI	0.7068
Pre- vs. post-IBT	TRQ	0.1895
Pre- vs. post-CGT	THI	0.5541
Pre- vs. post-CGT	TFI	0.1052
Pre-CGT vs. pre-IBT	THI	0.1451
Pre-CGT vs. pre-IBT	TFI	0.02505
Post-CGT vs. post-IBT	THI	0.3156
Post-CGT vs. post-IBT	TFI	0.6432

Cohen's d was calculated based on the THI, TFI, and TRQ scores at pre-IBT vs. post-IBT and at pre-CGT vs. post-CGT to show the effect size of the treatment on tinnitus. Cohen's d was also calculated for the THI and TFI scores at pre-CBT vs. pre-IBT and at post-CBT vs. post-IBT to highlight any potential baseline disparities between the control and case cohorts. A Cohen's d of 0.2 indicates a small effect size, 0.5 a medium effect size, and 0.8 a large effect size. IBT: Internet-based treatment; THI: Tinnitus Handicap Inventory; TFI: Tinnitus Functional Index; TRQ: Tinnitus Reactions Questionnaire; CGT: control group treatment.

Cohen's d was also calculated for patients who did not receive IBT (case control group, CGT), resulting in 0.55 for THI variation and 0.11 for TFI. This indicates a moderate effect on THI score and almost no effect on TFI. Cohen's d calculation was not performed in the CGT due to the limited sample size. Cohen's d calculation was also used to examine potential baseline disparities between the control and case cohorts, aiming to elucidate the impact of IBT. Among patients monitored using the THI, Cohen's d between cases and control was 0.15 at pre-treatment, while for those monitored with TFI, it was 0.03. These data show no baseline differences. Cohen's d calculation among the IBT group and CGT are shown in Table 1, demonstrating a difference in outcomes among the groups at the end of treatment, which is low-to-moderate for THI and moderate for TFI.

4. Discussion

This systematic review and meta-analysis aimed to investigate the efficacy of internet-based therapies for patients with tinnitus. The management of tinnitus primarily involves identifying and treating any underlying organic causes. However, in most cases, the origin of tinnitus remains unknown, necessitating a focus on reducing the intensity of the symptom and the associated distress. For acute tinnitus, particularly when linked to sudden hearing loss, current guidelines recommend systemic or intratympanic corticosteroid therapy [34]. In the case of chronic tinnitus without an identifiable cause, various treatment options exist, though the supporting evidence is often limited. The clinical efficacy and safety of repetitive transcranial magnetic stimulation (rTMS) in chronic tinnitus have been studied, but results are frequently divergent and sometimes contradictory, highlighting the need for further research in this area [2]. Sound therapy is another treatment often considered, since there have been no associated adverse effects, even though evidence for sound therapy as an effective solo treatment is inconclusive [2,35]. CBT stands out as the only treatment with moderate- to high-quality evidence supporting its efficacy [2]. However, CBT also presents some limitations associated with low patient compliance. For this reason, therapies administered via the internet have gain interest. Our results revealed a significant improvement in tinnitus severity and quality of life among patients who underwent internet-based therapies compared to treatments such as cognitive behavioral therapy, discussion forum, and face-to-face therapy.

Given the challenges in objectifying symptoms like tinnitus, THI, TFI, and TRQ questionnaires were used to assess both the subjectivity of the symptom and the efficacy of the treatment. More precisely, TRQ focuses on analyzing psychological distress, THI describes the impact of tinnitus on daily living, while TFI is validated to assess both the severity of tinnitus and measure treatment-related changes [9]. Our data highlighted that IBT positively impacted both THI and TFI (Cohen's d pre- vs. post-IBT was, respectively, 0.85 and 0.71). This indicates that IBT had a high positive impact on everyday life, as reflected in the decrease in THI scores. Furthermore, the decrease in TFI scores suggests a moderate to high efficacy of IBT in treating symptoms of tinnitus. On the other hand, TRQ showed a low decrease in scores, which could be attributed to the fact that only two studies using TRQ were considered for the analysis. When available, data on tinnitus status at the 1-year follow-up were considered to determine the long-term efficacy of IBT. Compared to the end of treatment, at the 1-year follow-up, TFI increased by one point, and THI increased by 5.77 points. This slight increase in scores at the 1-year follow-up compared to those immediately after therapy could be explained by a greater short-term effect compared to the long term. Overall, the total case population sustained improvements over time compared to the beginning of therapy, albeit with a slight decline compared to the immediate post-treatment period.

Finally, a few more considerations can be made when comparing the IBT group and CGT. Considering that TFI and THI scores were almost overlapping pre-treatment among cases and controls (Cohen's d lower than 0.2), there is a difference in the improvement of THI and TFI scores after treatment, with better results in the IBT group. Specifically, when comparing the IBT group with CGT, at the end of the treatment, the variations in THI and TFI describe a low–moderate difference in the subjective perception of tinnitus and a moderate difference in the efficacy of the treatment, respectively, highlighting better outcomes in the IBT group. These results could be attributed to better patient compliance resulting from the accessibility, cost-effectiveness, and customization of IBT.

While the number of available reviews is limited, our study aligns with existing literature, showing promise for future treatments. For instance, Beukes et al. [32] conducted a review specifically on internet-delivered cognitive behavioral therapy for tinnitus patients, finding a significant preference for Internet-based interventions over both inactive and active controls. Another systematic review by Demoen et al. [36] demonstrated low to moderate evidence of reduced tinnitus severity and distress in patients treated with telerehabilitation. However, high dropout rates due to factors like lack of time, engagement, motivation, and patient openness were noted, leading to concerns about bias and certainty levels. A slightly different conclusion was drawn from the systematic review conducted by Nagaraj et al. [4], which focused on internet- and smartphone-based applications for treating tinnitus. Their analysis revealed a comparable improvement in both traditional and internet-delivered forms of tinnitus treatment, highlighting their effectiveness. However, unlike previous studies, Nagaraj and colleagues did not find a significant difference in treatment outcomes for patients undergoing internet-delivered therapies than conventional ones. Moreover, various causes of tinnitus are described in the literature [5,37]. Some of these causes could be transient, a factor that should be considered when analyzing data regarding tinnitus. However, even if patients who would have naturally improved or recovered "on their own" were included in this analysis, our findings still demonstrate a better outcome in patients undergoing IBT compared to the CGT.

IBTs hold promise in overcoming some of the limitations associated with conventional therapies, ensuring accessibility, cost reduction, and consequently enhancing patient compliance. More precisely, from a practical and economic perspective, the cost of management is a significant consideration for many patients with tinnitus. In countries with insurance-based healthcare systems, tinnitus management is often not covered by many insurance companies. Thus, the accessibility of internet-based therapies represents an important advancement in providing a non-invasive, supportive, and more affordable method of tinnitus management. Furthermore, given the easy accessibility associated with IBTs, these technologies could achieve widespread adoption among patients. This widespread use has the potential to significantly improve the quality of life for a large number of individuals, ultimately resulting in a more productive and functional role for patients in society.

A few considerations should be made about the limitations of this meta-analysis. First, the heterogeneity of treatment observed within both the patient and control groups presents a challenge. The meta-analysis intentionally did not focus on the comparison of a specific internet-based therapy with its face-to-face counterpart but rather sought to examine the overall efficacy of IBTs without focusing on specific modalities. The goal of this meta-analysis was indeed to assess the efficacy and reach of digital interventions as a whole. This certainly represents a limitation, but at the same time it could be considered as a direction for future studies. Despite the utilization of standardized questionnaires, the subjective nature of tinnitus symptoms and individual variations in response to it represent an element that is not easily standardizable into a meta-analysis. Furthermore, the small sample size hindered our ability to conduct uniform statistical analyses across all the groups of patients monitored with different questionnaires. This limitation underscores the need for larger and more diverse datasets to provide more robust conclusions in future studies. This approach would help identify the most suitable therapy to improve the quality of life of patients with tinnitus. Finally, exploring the variables that influence patient compliance and the adoption of IBTs could provide further insights into how to optimize these therapies for greater economic and therapeutic impact.

5. Conclusions

Despite improvements observed in patients undergoing therapies such as CBT, discussion forum, and face-to-face therapy, internet-based treatments have demonstrated reliable effectiveness in significantly reducing THI and TFI scores. This suggests that internet-based therapies offer a promising avenue for enhancing tinnitus management strategies, ensuring accessibility, reducing costs, and consequently improving patient compliance.

Author Contributions: Conceptualization, M.A.; methodology, E.S. and M.A.; software, E.S. and K.C.; validation, G.T., A.G. and M.A.; formal analysis, E.S.; investigation, K.C. and C.A.M.; resources, K.C. and C.A.M.; data curation, E.S. and C.A.M.; writing—original draft preparation, E.S. and C.A.M.;

writing—review and editing, G.T., A.G. and M.A.; supervision, M.A. All authors have read and agreed to the published version of the manuscript.

Funding: M.A. was supported by the National Center for Research Resources and the National Center for Advancing Translational Sciences, National Institutes of Health, via Grant TL1TR001415.

Institutional Review Board Statement: Ethical review and approval were waived for this study because it consists of a systematic review of the literature. No human subjects or animals were directly involved. All the included data were already published in the literature.

Informed Consent Statement: Patient consent was waived because this is a systematic review of the literature, and no human subjects or animals were directly involved. The included data were already published in the literature.

Data Availability Statement: The data that support the findings of this study are available from the corresponding authors upon reasonable request.

Conflicts of Interest: The authors declare no conflicts of interest.

Appendix A

List of exact search terms used in each database.

PubMed Search. Search: (((Tinnitus[mh] OR Tinnitus[tiab]) AND (Therapy/Narrow[filter])) OR ((Tinnitus[mh] OR Tinnitus[tiab]) AND (Random*[tiab] OR RCT[tiab]))) AND (Smartphone OR "smart phone*" OR handheld computer OR Internet OR Mobile Device OR Tablet Computer OR Mobile Applications OR mobile app OR Telemedicine OR Online OR Virtual Medicine OR Telehealth OR eHealth OR Telecare OR Mobile Health OR mHealth OR virtualHealth OR "Virtual Health" OR virtual visit* OR Distance Counseling OR Telepathology OR Telerehabilitation OR E-therapy OR E-Counseling OR Virtual Healthcare)

Scopus Search. Tinnitus AND (Smartphone OR "smart phone*" OR "handheld computer" OR Internet OR "Mobile Device" OR Tablet OR "Mobile Application*" OR "mobile app" OR Telemedicine OR Online OR Virtual* OR Telehealth OR eHealth OR Telecare OR "Mobile Health" OR mHealth OR "Distance Counseling" OR Telepathology OR Telerehabilitation OR "E therapy" OR "E Counseling")

Cochrane CENTRAL. 121 Trials matching tinnitus in Title Abstract Keyword AND (Smartphone OR "smart phone" OR handheld computer OR Internet OR Mobile Device OR Tablet Computer OR Mobile Applications OR mobile app OR Telemedicine OR Online OR Virtual Medicine OR Telehealth OR eHealth OR Telecare OR Mobile Health OR mHealth OR virtualHealth OR "Virtual Health" OR virtual visit* OR Distance Counseling OR Telepathology OR Telerehabilitation OR E-therapy OR E-Counseling OR Virtual Healthcare) in Title Abstract Keyword–(Word variations have been searched)

Web of Science Core Collection. Tinnitus AND (Smartphone OR "smart phone*" OR "handheld computer" OR Internet OR "Mobile Device" OR Tablet OR "Mobile Application*" OR "mobile app" OR Telemedicine OR Online OR Virtual* OR Telehealth OR eHealth OR Telecare OR "Mobile Health" OR mHealth OR "Distance Counseling" OR Telepathology OR Telerehabilitation OR "E therapy" OR "E Counseling") (All Fields) and Random* OR RCT (All Fields) and Article (Document Types)

Appendix B

Table A1. Characteristics of the included studies.

uthor	Year of Publication	Country of Cohort	Total Number of Patients	Number of Case Group Patients	Modality of Treatment	Type of Treatment in Case Groups	Type of Treatment in Control Groups (if RCT)	Time of Treatment (Weeks)	Questionnaire Used
Veise	2016	Germany	124	62	PC	iCBT	DF	8	THI
Kim	2017	Korea	26	26	Smartphone	Music		12	THI

Table A1. *Cont.*

Author	Year of Publication	Country of Cohort	Total Number of Patients	Number of Case Group Patients	Modality of Treatment	Type of Treatment in Case Groups	Type of Treatment in Control Groups (if RCT)	Time of Treatment (Weeks)	Questionnaire Used
Rheker	2015	Germany	112	56	Person	iCBT + therapist	iCBT	8	THI
Beukes	2022	USA	200	200	PC	iCBT		8	TFI
Kaldo	2013	Sweden	293	293	PC	iCBT		8	TRQ
Kaldo	2008	Sweden	51	26	PC	iCBT	CBT	8	TRQ
				26	PC	iCBT	CBT	8	THI
Jasper	2014	Germany		41	PC	iCBT	CBT	10	THI
				41	PC	iCBT	DF	10	THI
Hesser	2012	Sweden	99	32	PC	iCBT	DF	8	THI
				35	PC	ACT	DF	8	THI
Beukes	2018	UK	146	73	PC	iCBT	DF	8	TFI
Beukes	2018	UK	92	46	PC	iCBT	F2F	8	TFI
									THI
Beukes	2021	USA	27	27	PC	iCBT		8	TFI
Abouzari	2021	USA	30	20	Smartphone	iCBT + sound therapy	DF	8	THI
Beukes	2017	UK	37	37	PC	iCBT + therapist		8	TFI
Malinvaud	2016	France	148	61	PC	Virtual reality	CBT	12	THI

RCT: randomized control trial; iCBT: internet-based cognitive behavioral therapy; CBT: cognitive behavioral therapy; DF: discussion forum; ACT: acceptance and commitment therapy; F2F: face-to-face; THI: Tinnitus Handicap Inventory; TFI: Tinnitus Functional Index; TRQ: Tinnitus Reaction Questionnaire.

Appendix C

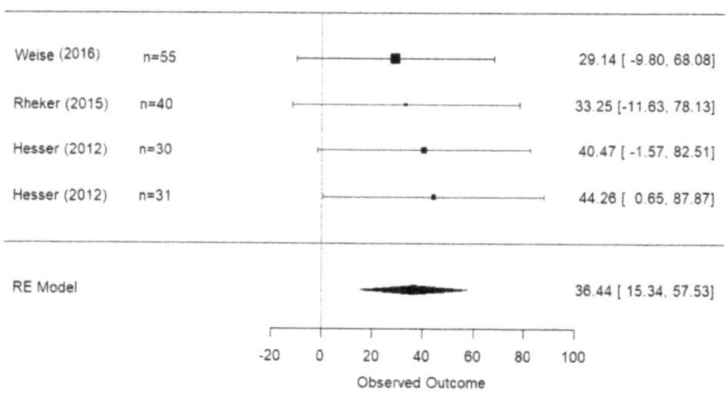

Figure A1. THI at 12-month follow-up in Internet-based treatment group [26,31,32].

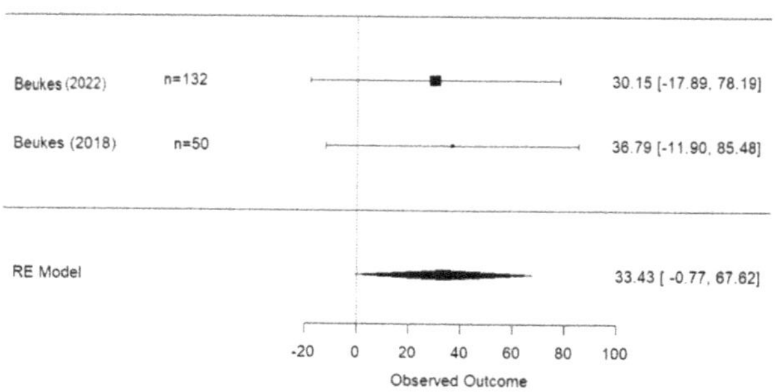

Figure A2. TFI at 12-month follow-up in in Internet-based treatment group [22,23].

erences

Noreña, A.J.; Lacher-Fougère, S.; Fraysse, M.-J.; Bizaguet, E.; Grevin, P.; Thai-Van, H.; Moati, L.; Le Pajolec, C.; Fournier, P.; Ohresser, M.; et al. Chapter 21—A contribution to the debate on tinnitus definition. In *Progress in Brain Research*; Langguth, B., Kleinjung, T., De Ridder, D., Schlee, W., Vanneste, S., Eds.; Elsevier: Amsterdam, The Netherlands, 2021; Volume 262, pp. 469–485. [CrossRef]

Dalrymple, S.N.; Lewis, S.H.; Philman, S. Tinnitus: Diagnosis and Management. *Am. Fam. Physician* **2021**, *103*, 663–671. [PubMed]

Jarach, C.M.; Lugo, A.; Scala, M.; van den Brandt, P.A.; Cederroth, C.R.; Odone, A.; Garavello, W.; Schlee, W.; Langguth, B.; Gallus, S. Global Prevalence and Incidence of Tinnitus: A Systematic Review and Meta-analysis. *JAMA Neurol.* **2022**, *79*, 888–900. [CrossRef] [PubMed]

Nagaraj, M.K.; Prabhu, P. Internet/smartphone-based applications for the treatment of tinnitus: A systematic review. *Eur. Arch. Otorhinolaryngol.* **2020**, *277*, 649–657. [CrossRef] [PubMed]

Baguley, D.; McFerran, D.; Hall, D. Tinnitus. *Lancet* **2013**, *382*, 1600–1607. [CrossRef] [PubMed]

Narsinh, K.H.; Hui, F.; Saloner, D.; Tu-Chan, A.; Sharon, J.; Rauschecker, A.M.; Safoora, F.; Shah, V.; Meisel, K.; Amans, M.R. Diagnostic Approach to Pulsatile Tinnitus: A Narrative Review. *JAMA Otolaryngol. Head Neck Surg.* **2022**, *148*, 476. [CrossRef]

van der Wal, A.; Michiels, S.; Van de Heyning, P.; Braem, M.; Visscher, C.M.; Topsakal, V.; Gilles, A.; Jacquemin, L.; Van Rompaey, V.; De Hertogh, W. Treatment of Somatosensory Tinnitus: A Randomized Controlled Trial Studying the Effect of Orofacial Treatment as Part of a Multidisciplinary Program. *J. Clin. Med.* **2020**, *9*, 705. [CrossRef] [PubMed]

Benjamin, T.; Gillard, D.; Abouzari, M.; Djalilian, H.R.; Sharon, J.D. Vestibular and Auditory Manifestations of Migraine. *Curr. Opin. Neurol.* **2022**, *35*, 84–89. [CrossRef] [PubMed]

Theodoroff, S.M. Tinnitus Questionnaires for Research and Clinical Use. In *The Behavioral Neuroscience of Tinnitus*; Searchfield, G.D., Zhang, J., Eds.; Springer International Publishing: Cham, Germany, 2021; pp. 403–418. [CrossRef]

Wilson, P.H.; Henry, J.; Bowen, M.; Haralambous, G. Tinnitus reaction questionnaire: Psychometric properties of a measure of distress associated with tinnitus. *J. Speech Hear. Res.* **1991**, *34*, 197–201. [CrossRef]

Newman, C.W.; Jacobson, G.P.; Spitzer, J.B. Development of the Tinnitus Handicap Inventory. *Arch. Otolaryngol. Head Neck Surg.* **1996**, *122*, 143–148. [CrossRef] [PubMed]

Meikle, M.B.; Henry, J.A.; Griest, S.E.; Stewart, B.J.; Abrams, H.B.; McArdle, R.; Myers, P.J.; Newman, C.W.; Sandridge, S.; Turk, D.C.; et al. The Tinnitus Functional Index: Development of a New Clinical Measure for Chronic, Intrusive Tinnitus. *Ear Hear.* **2012**, *33*, 153–176. [CrossRef]

Mazurek, B.; Böcking, B.; Dobel, C.; Rose, M.; Brüggemann, P. Tinnitus und beeinflussende Komorbiditäten. *Laryngorhinootologie* **2023**, *102*, S50–S58. [CrossRef] [PubMed]

Henry, J.A. Sound Therapy to Reduce Auditory Gain for Hyperacusis and Tinnitus. *Am. J. Audiol.* **2022**, *31*, 1067–1077. [CrossRef] [PubMed]

Liang, Z.; Yang, H.; Cheng, G.; Huang, L.; Zhang, T.; Jia, H. Repetitive transcranial magnetic stimulation on chronic tinnitus: A systematic review and meta-analysis. *BMC Psychiatry* **2020**, *20*, 547. [CrossRef]

Martins, M.L.; da Silva Souza, D.; Cavalcante, M.E.D.O.B.; Barboza, H.N.; de Medeiros, J.F.; Dos Santos Andrade, S.M.M.; da Silva Machado, D.G.; da Rosa, M.R.D. Effect of transcranial Direct Current Stimulation for tinnitus treatment: A systematic review and meta-analysis. *Neurophysiol. Clin.* **2022**, *52*, 1–16. [CrossRef] [PubMed]

Basner, L.; Smit, J.V.; Zeitler, D.M.; Schwartz, S.R.; Krause, K.; Bansal, A.; Farrokhi, F. Deep Brain Stimulation for Primary Refractory Tinnitus: A Systematic Review. *Brain Sci.* **2024**, *14*, 452. [CrossRef]

Normand, S.-L.T. Meta-analysis: Formulating, evaluating, combining, and reporting. *Stat. Med.* **1999**, *18*, 321–359. [CrossRef]

Searchfield, G.D.; Sanders, P.J. A randomized single-blind controlled trial of a prototype digital polytherapeutic for tinnitus. *Front. Neurol.* **2022**, *13*, 958730. [CrossRef] [PubMed]

Abouzari, M.; Goshtasbi, K.; Sarna, B.; Ghavami, Y.; Parker, E.M.; Khosravi, P.; Mostaghni, N.; Jamshidi, S.; Saber, T.; Djalilian, H.R. Adapting Personal Therapies Using a Mobile Application for Tinnitus Rehabilitation: A Preliminary Study. *Ann. Otol. Rhinol. Laryngol.* **2021**, *130*, 571–577. [CrossRef]

Beukes, E.W.; Andersson, G.; Manchaiah, V. Long-term efficacy of audiologist-guided Internet-based cognitive behaviour therapy for tinnitus in the United States: A repeated-measures design. *Internet Interv.* **2022**, *30*, 100583. [CrossRef] [PubMed]

Beukes, E.W.; Allen, P.M.; Baguley, D.M.; Manchaiah, V.; Andersson, G. Long-Term Efficacy of Audiologist-Guided Internet-Based Cognitive Behavior Therapy for Tinnitus. *Am. J. Audiol.* **2018**, *27*, 431–447. [CrossRef]

Beukes, E.W.; Andersson, G.; Allen, P.M.; Manchaiah, V.; Baguley, D.M. Effectiveness of Guided Internet-Based Cognitive Behavioral Therapy vs Face-to-Face Clinical Care for Treatment of Tinnitus: A Randomized Clinical Trial. *JAMA Otolaryngol. Head Neck Surg.* **2018**, *144*, 1126. [CrossRef] [PubMed]

Beukes, E.W.; Andersson, G.; Fagelson, M.; Manchaiah, V. Audiologist-Supported Internet-Based Cognitive Behavioral Therapy for Tinnitus in the United States: A Pilot Trial. *Am. J. Audiol.* **2021**, *30*, 717–729. [CrossRef]

Hesser, H.; Gustafsson, T.; Lundén, C.; Henrikson, O.; Fattahi, K.; Johnsson, E.; Westin, V.Z.; Carlbring, P.; Maki-Torkko, E.; Kaldo, V.; et al. A randomized controlled trial of internet-delivered cognitive behavior therapy and acceptance and commitment therapy in the treatment of tinnitus. *J. Consult. Clin. Psychol.* **2012**, *80*, 649–661. [CrossRef] [PubMed]

26. Jasper, K.; Weise, C.; Conrad, I.; Andersson, G.; Hiller, W.; Kleinstäuber, M. Internet-Based Guided Self-Help versus Gr Cognitive Behavioral Therapy for Chronic Tinnitus: A Randomized Controlled Trial. *Psychother. Psychosom.* **2014**, *83*, 234– [CrossRef] [PubMed]
27. Kaldo, V.; Haak, T.; Buhrman, M.; Alfonsson, S.; Larsen, H.-C.; Andersson, G. Internet-Based Cognitive Behaviour Therapy Tinnitus Patients Delivered in a Regular Clinical Setting: Outcome and Analysis of Treatment Dropout. *Cogn. Behav. Ther.* **2** *42*, 146–158. [CrossRef]
28. Kaldo, V.; Levin, S.; Widarsson, J.; Buhrman, M.; Larsen, H.-C.; Andersson, G. Internet Versus Group Cognitive-Behavi Treatment of Distress Associated With Tinnitus: A Randomized Controlled Trial. *Behav. Ther.* **2008**, *39*, 348–359. [Cross [PubMed]
29. Kim, S.Y.; Chang, M.Y.; Hong, M.; Yoo, S.-G.; Oh, D.; Park, M.K. Tinnitus therapy using tailor-made notched music delive via a smartphone application and Ginko combined treatment: A pilot study. *Auris Nasus Larynx* **2017**, *44*, 528–533. [Cross [PubMed]
30. Rheker, J.; Andersson, G.; Weise, C. The role of "on demand" therapist guidance vs. no support in the treatment of tinnitus the internet: A randomized controlled trial. *Internet Interv.* **2015**, *2*, 189–199. [CrossRef]
31. Weise, C.; Kleinstäuber, M.; Andersson, G. Internet-Delivered Cognitive-Behavior Therapy for Tinnitus: A Randomized Contro Trial. *Psychosom. Med.* **2016**, *78*, 501–510. [CrossRef]
32. Beukes, E.W.; Allen, P.M.; Manchaiah, V.; Baguley, D.M.; Andersson, G. Internet-Based Intervention for Tinnitus: Outcome Single-Group Open Trial. *J. Am. Acad. Audiol.* **2017**, *28*, 340–351. [CrossRef]
33. Malinvaud, D.; Londero, A.; Niarra, R.; Peignard, P.; Warusfel, O.; Viaud-Delmon, I.; Chatellier, G.; Bonfils, P. Auditory and vi 3D virtual reality therapy as a new treatment for chronic subjective tinnitus: Results of a randomized controlled trial. *Hear.* **2016**, *333*, 127–135. [CrossRef] [PubMed]
34. Mazurek, B.; Hesse, G.; Dobel, C.; Kratzsch, V.; Lahmann, C.; Sattel, H. *Clinical Practice Guideline: Chronic Tinnitus—Diagnosis Treatment*; Deutsches Ärzteblatt International: Cologne, Germany, 2022. [CrossRef]
35. Brennan-Jones, C.G.; Thomas, A.; Hoare, D.J.; Sereda, M. Cochrane corner: Sound therapy (using amplification devices and sound generators) for tinnitus. *Int. J. Audiol.* **2020**, *59*, 161–165. [CrossRef] [PubMed]
36. Demoen, S.; Chalimourdas, A.; Timmermans, A.; Van Rompaey, V.; Vanderveken, O.M.; Jacquemin, L.; Schlee, W.; Marneffe, Luyten, J.; Gilles, A.; et al. Effectiveness of Telerehabilitation Interventions for Self-management of Tinnitus: Systematic Rev *J. Med. Internet Res.* **2023**, *25*, e39076. [CrossRef] [PubMed]
37. Langrodi, S.S.R.; Goudarzi, F.; Stanbouly, D. Etiology of Tinnitus on CT and CBCT: A Narrative Review. *Int. Tinnitus J.* **2022** 95–100. [CrossRef]

Journal of
*Personalized
Medicine*

MDPI

cle

ıin after Licorice or Sugar-Water Gargling in Patients ecovering from Oropharyngeal Surgery—A Randomized, ouble-Blind Trial

ita Windpassinger [1,2,*], Michal Prusak [1], Jana Gemeiner [1], Olga Plattner [1,2], Stefan Janik [3], Gerold Besser [3], lfgang Gstoettner [3], Pu Xuan [4,5], Daniel I. Sessler [2,6] and Kurt Ruetzler [2,5,7]

1 Department of Anesthesia, Critical Care and Pain Medicine, Division of General Anesthesia and Intensive Care Medicine, Medical University Vienna, 1090 Vienna, Austria
2 Outcomes Research Consortium, Houston, TX 77030, USA; ds@or.org (D.I.S.); kr@or.org (K.R.)
3 Department of Otorhinolaryngology, Medical University Vienna, 1090 Vienna, Austria
4 Department of Quantitative Health Sciences, Cleveland Clinics, Cleveland, OH 44195, USA
5 Department of Outcomes Research, Cleveland Clinics, Cleveland, OH 44195, USA
6 Department of Anesthesiology and Center for Outcomes Research, University of Texas Health Science Center, Houston, TX 77030, USA
7 Department of General Anesthesiology, Anesthesiology Institute, Cleveland Clinics, Cleveland, OH 44195, USA
* Correspondence: marita.windpassinger@meduniwien.ac.at; Tel.: +43-1-40400-41020

Abstract: Background: Glycyrrhiza glabrata (licorice) is used in traditional medicine and herbal remedies and reduces sore throats consequent to intubation, but whether it is protective for more intense pain after oropharyngeal surgery remains unclear. We thus tested the joint hypothesis that gargling with licorice, which has anti-inflammatory and antioxidant properties, reduces postoperative pain and morphine consumption. Methods: We enrolled patients having elective oropharyngeal surgery. Participants were randomly allocated to gargle with either 1 g licorice or a sugar placebo before and for up to three days after surgery. A numerical rating scale (NRS) for pain along with morphine consumption was evaluated every 30 min during the post-anesthesia care unit (PACU) stay and then three times daily for three days. We pre-specified that licorice gargling would be deemed better than sugar gargling only if found non-inferior on both morphine consumption and pain score and superior on at least one of the two. Results: 65 patients were randomized to the licorice group and 61 to placebo. We found noninferiority (NI) in pain scores with an estimated mean difference of −0.09 (95.2% CI: −0.88, 0.70; $p = 0.001$; NI delta = 1) between licorice and placebo gargling. There were no adverse events reported in either group that required treatment discontinuation. Conclusions: Gargling with licorice did not significantly or meaningfully reduce postoperative pain or morphine consumption in patients recovering from oropharyngeal surgery. While higher doses might prove more effective, our results suggest that other topical analgesics should be considered.

Keywords: anesthesia; licorice; postoperative pain; analgesia; oropharyngeal surgery; gargling; pain management

1. Introduction

Postoperative pain is a major cause of patient dissatisfaction [1]. Severe pain and difficulty in swallowing that compromise food intake are common in patients recovering from oropharyngeal surgery, and both impair well-being and sleep [2,3]. For example, Coulthard et al. reported that 93% of patients after oral and maxillofacial surgery experienced postoperative pain, ranging from moderate (47%) to severe (34%) [4]. Effective acute analgesia may prevent central sensation and the development of prolonged pain states. Pain is therefore a substantial issue for a large proportion of patients recovering from oral and maxillofacial surgery.

Topical treatments have the advantage of avoiding systemic effects, especially those caused by opioids. Various types of mouthwash and topical analgesic sprays reduce postoperative throat pain [5–8]. Gargling with an analgesic solution, for example, provides topical pain relief [9–12]. Postoperative licorice gargling is a well-documented method of preventing sore throats subsequent to intubation. Two trials each report that licorice reduces post-intubation sore throat, hoarseness, and coughing by a factor of two [13,14].

Licorice is a unique-tasting herb derived from glycyrrhiza glabra that contains various active ingredients, the most important of which are glycyrrhizic acid, glycyrrhizin, liquilitin, liquiritigeninglabridin, and hispaglabridins [15,16]. Glycyrrhizic acid is the main active ingredient in licorice root, and it is a triterpenoid saponin. It is a natural sweetener and flavoring agent commonly used in food and beverages, as well as in traditional medicine. Glycyrrhizic acid has various pharmacological effects, including anti-inflammation via inhibition of cyclooxygenase activity, prostaglandin formation, and platelet aggregation [17].

Glycyrrhetic acid is a metabolite of glycyrrhizic acid, formed by enzymatic cleavage of glycyrrhizic acid in the body. It is pharmacologically similar to glycyrrhizic acid and has similar anti-inflammatory, antioxidant and antiviral effects. Its other pharmacological activities include inhibiting type two 11-beta-hydroxysteroid dehydrogenase, which causes a cortisol-induced mineralocorticoid reaction [18]. Consequently, glycyrrhizin inhibits the production of pro-inflammatory cytokines and chemokines, which are involved in the initiation and progression of inflammatory processes [19]. Licorice flavonoids, such as liquiritigenin and isoliquiritigenin, also exhibit anti-inflammatory activity through the suppression of the nuclear factor kappa B pathway, which is involved in the regulation of immune responses and inflammation. Other anti-inflammatory properties include reduced expression of tumor necrosis factor-α, interleukin-6, inducible nitric oxidase synthase, and cyclooxygenase-2 in animal models [20,21].

A recent study evaluated the dose-dependence of licorice on postoperative sore throat, concluding that analgesia is better with 1 g licorice than at lower doses [22]. However, pain after oral surgery is far more intense than that from laryngoscopy and intubation. Whether gargling with licorice provides adequate analgesia after oropharyngeal surgery remains unknown. We therefore tested the joint primary hypotheses that gargling with 1 g licorice reduces pain scores and decreases morphine better than gargling with sugar water in patients recovering from elective oropharyngeal surgeries.

2. Materials and Methods

This trial was approved by the Medical University of Vienna Institutional Review Board (IRB #1308/2016), and written informed consent was obtained from all subjects participating in the trial. The trial was registered prior to patient enrollment at clinicaltrials.gov (NCT 02968823, Principal investigator: Olga Plattner MD, Date of registration: 16 November 2016).

2.1. Subject Selection

We enrolled children and adults between the ages of 12 and 99 years who were scheduled for elective oropharyngeal surgeries at the Department of Otorhinolaryngology in the Medical University Vienna, Austria. Legal guardians consented on behalf of patients <18 years old; patients 16–17 years old also assented; and patients ≥18 years old consented.

We included patients who had an American Society of Anesthesiologists (ASA) physical status 1–3. Elective oropharyngeal surgeries included panendoscopic surgery with larynx intubation using a small endotracheal tube followed by the introduction of a rigid airway for patients with tumors in the pharyngeal, hypopharyngeal, or laryngeal area. Other surgeries included tonsillectomy-adenotonsillectomies or biopsies for suspected tongue carcinoma.

We excluded patients with known or suspected allergies to licorice or its components, insulin-dependent diabetes mellitus, liver disease, or liver failure with bleeding disorders. We also excluded patients who took non-steroidal anti-inflammatory drugs within 24 h before surgery, chronically used morphine, were unable to use an intravenous patient-controlled analgesia pump, had a severely infected oropharyngeal tumor, required rapid sequence induction, or were expected to need mechanical ventilation after surgery.

2.2. Protocol

Participating patients were randomly assigned to gargle with licorice solution or placebo. Randomization was based on computer-generated codes with random blocking and no stratification. Assignments were kept in sequentially numbered opaque envelopes that were opened shortly before surgery. Allocation was thus concealed as long as practical.

The licorice solution consisted of 1 g licorice (extractum liquiritiae fluidum) diluted in 30 mL of water. The placebo solution was 5 g sugar, also diluted in 30 mL water, an amount that is comparably sweet. The solutions were kept in identical-looking bottles. Patients were asked to gargle with the trial solution for 60 s without swallowing, under the supervision and direct observation of an investigator not subsequently involved in data collection. Gargling was repeated two hours postoperatively and then three times daily for three days while patients remained hospitalized. As practical, gargling was timed to 30 min before eating. Patients, clinicians, and investigators were blinded to all treatments. Participating patients were told that two comparably sweet solutions were used for this trial but were not told what flavors were being tested or the trial hypothesis.

General anesthesia was induced with propofol (3–5 mg kg^{-1}), fentanyl (3–5 μg kg^{-1}) and rocuronium (0.6 mg kg^{-1}) for muscle relaxation, and anesthesia was maintained with remifentanil 0.15–0.4 μg/kg/min and propofol 3–5 mg/kg/h. The trachea was gently intubated with a flexible tube size of 6–6.5 mm inner diameter for women and 7–7.5 mm inner diameter for men. Anesthetic administration was titrated to target a Narcotrend range between 40 and 55 (MonitorTechnik, Bad Bramdstedt, Germany) and to mean arterial pressure within 20% of pre-induction values. Mechanical ventilation with an oxygen-air mixture was adjusted to maintain end-tidal PCO_2 between 32 and 35 mmHg as clinically practical.

Before transfer to the post-anesthesia care unit (PACU), patients were connected to an intravenous patient-controlled-analgesia (PCA) pump, starting with a bolus of 2 mg morphine hydrochloride at initiation of PCA, followed by demand doses of 2 mg with a lockout interval of 10 min and an hourly limit of 12 mg. A single dose of 500 mg metamizole IV (or paracetamol 500 mg in patients allergic to metamizole) was given during surgery. An additional dose was given in the PACU if necessary. Thereafter, pain was treated with morphine hydrochloride boluses per PCA until the first postoperative day, when patients were transitioned to oral metamizole, paracetamol, and dexibuprofen as necessary. Patients stayed at least one night in the hospital. They were discharged home with a supply of metamizole 500 mg tablets and dexibuprofen 400 mg tablets for analgesia.

2.3. Measurements

Demographic and morphometric characteristics, including sex, age, body weight, height, ASA Physical Status, and Mallampati Score were recorded. Anesthetic and surgical characteristics included type of surgery and total amounts of propofol, remifentanil, and fentanyl. Pain scores, incidence of coughing, and overall analgesic consumption during the initial three days after surgery were observed.

Patients were asked to record the severity of pain, cough intensity, adverse effects, and pain medications three times daily on each of the initial 3 postoperative days. Verbal pain scores were based on a Likert scale from 0 to 10, with 0 signifying no pain and 10 signifying the worst imaginable pain. Pain scores were recorded immediately after tracheal extubation every 30 min in the PACU for the first 2 h, on surgical wards 1 h after gargling, and then daily for up to 3 postoperative days at home. Other outcome assessments included coughing intensity (rated as none, mild, moderate, or severe) at 30, 60, 90, and 120 min after arrival in the PACU.

2.4. Statistical Methods

Demographic characteristics, including age, sex, weight, and race, ASA physical status, Mallampati score, surgery type, and intraoperative anesthetic variables, are summarized in Table 1. Baseline variables with an absolute standardized difference (ASD) > 0.349 (i.e., $1.96\times\sqrt{\frac{1}{n_1}+\frac{1}{n_2}}$), where n_1 and n_2 are the number of patients in each group, were considered imbalanced and adjusted for in all analyses. Analyses were conducted based on a modified intent-to-treat basis where we included all randomized patients who received the treatment at least once.

Table 1. Baseline and demographic characteristics.

	Sugar (n = 61)	Licorice (n = 65)	ASD
Age, years	37 ± 18	43 ± 19	0.306
Female	25 (41)	31 (48)	0.135
White	60 (98)	65 (100)	0.183
Weight, kg	75 ± 17	74 ± 15	0.036
Height, cm	172 ± 9	171 ± 10	0.116
ASA status, n, %			0.468
1	41 (67)	29 (45)	
2	17 (28)	31 (48)	
3	3 (5)	5 (8)	
Mallampati score			0.345
1	40 (66)	35 (54)	
2	19 (31)	23 (35)	
3	2 (3)	6 (9)	
4	0 (0.0)	1 (2)	
Type of surgery			0.524
Pan-Endoscopy	17 (28)	30 (46)	
Tonsillectomy/Adenotonsillectomy	41 (67)	34 (52)	
Biopsy/demarcation of Ca of tongue	0 (0.0)	1 (2)	
Other	3 (5)	0 (0.0)	
Preoperative pain score	0.31 ± 0.87	0.37 ± 1.17	0.054
Intraoperative			
Propofol, mg	450 [360, 590]	385 [304, 515]	0.228
Remifentanil, mg	820 [461, 1000]	719 [500, 1000]	0.052
Fentanyl, mg	150 [100, 200]	150 [100, 200]	0.115
Metamizole, mg	1.00 [1.00, 1.00]	1.00 [1.00, 1.00]	0.008
Immediate cough after surgery			0.323
0	44 (72)	54 (83)	
1	13 (21)	7 (11)	
2	3 (5)	2 (3)	
3	1 (2)	2 (3)	

Variables are presented as means ± SDs, counts (percent), or medians [Q1, Q3] appropriately. ASA physical status: American Society of Anesthesiologists physical status. ASD: absolute standardized difference, defined as difference in means of proportions divided by pooled standard deviation. Baseline variables with absolute standardized difference (ASD) > 0.349 (i.e., $1.96\times\sqrt{\frac{1}{n_1}+\frac{1}{n_2}}$) were considered imbalanced.

2.4.1. Primary Analysis

The primary outcomes were total morphine consumption and pain scores at rest during the first 2 h after the surgery. The effect of licorice gargling on pain scores and total morphine consumption during the first 2 h after arrival in PACU was assessed using a "joint hypothesis testing" framework. Using this framework, we pre-specified that licorice gargling would be deemed better than sugar gargling only if it was found to be non-inferior on both morphine consumption and pain score and superior on at least one of the two (Supplemental Figure S1).

We assessed the treatment effect on pain score over time in a repeated-measures linear model assuming autoregressive within-subject correlation structure. If there was a treatment-by-time interaction detected ($p < 0.10$), we would assess group differences at each measurement time. If the interaction was not significant, we would assess the group difference over all the measurements. We assessed the effect on morphine consumption in a linear regression model using log-transformed morphine consumption as the outcome, with the treatment effect expressed as a ratio of geometric means.

Using the estimated difference between licorice and sugar-water groups, noninferiority was tested using both the confidence interval method and a statistical test for noninferiority. Specifically, noninferiority would be claimed for morphine consumption if the upper limit of the 95% 2-sided confidence interval for the ratio of geometric means of total morphine consumption was less than the noninferiority delta of 1.15, and for pain if the difference in mean scores was less than the noninferiority delta of 1 (on our 11 point scale).

If noninferiority was claimed on both primary outcomes, superiority testing in the same direction would be conducted using the confidence interval method and statistical tests. Superiority would be claimed if the upper limit of the 97.5% confidence interval of the ratio of means was less than 1 for morphine consumption or if the 97.5% confidence interval of the pain score difference was less than 0 for pain scores.

2.4.2. Secondary Analysis

We did not analyze the amount of coughing in the PACU since coughing scores were all 1 or 0; thus, an analysis of coughing incidence was sufficient. For pain, we used a generalized linear mixed model with binomial distribution with logit link assuming a covariance type of variance components (VC) to account for within-subject correlation. For pain scores from the end of surgery until the first postoperative morning, pain scores during postoperative day 1 (POD1) up to postoperative day 3 (POD3), separate linear mixed models were used to estimate the treatment effect on each corresponding outcome, assuming an autoregressive correlation structure to account for within-subject correlation. For total morphine consumption until postoperative day 1 morning and pain medication during POD1-POD3, a separate generalized linear model with Gaussian distribution and identity link was used with log-transformation applied on each corresponding cumulative morphine consumption.

The significance level for joint hypothesis testing was 0.05 overall and thus 0.025 overall in one direction for the noninferiority and superiority tests. No adjustment for 2 noninferiority tests was needed since noninferiority was required on both primary outcomes (95% CI used for each noninferiority test). Bonferroni correction was used for superiority testing since significance on either outcome was sufficient (97.5% confidence interval CI used for superiority tests). The significance level was 0.024 for this final analysis for noninferiority testing after adjustment for the sequential design, specifically spending alpha of 0.001 at the first interim analysis). Thus, 95.2% confidence intervals were calculated for the noninferiority tests. The significance level was 0.05 overall for the two-sided tests in secondary analyses, and thus the significance criterion was 0.01 for each secondary analysis after Bonferroni correction for multiple testing (0.05/5 = 0.01).

2.5. Sample Size and Power

A total of 252 patients were needed to achieve 90% power to detect noninferiority on both pain score (noninferiority delta of 1 on a scale of 0–10) and total morphine consumption (noninferiority delta of 1.15) and superiority on either outcome at the overall 0.025 significance level, including 3 interim analyses. Power was estimated using the statistical software suite (SAS) macro (developed for designs with joint hypothesis testing) and the SAS Seq Design procedure. The power calculation was based on 1000 simulations, assuming a mean (SD) pain score of 2 (2) and 3 (2) for the licorice and the sugar-water groups, respectively, and a coefficient of variation (standard deviation SD/mean) for morphine consumption of 0.25 for both groups. For both outcomes, we assumed an autoregressive correlation structure with an adjacent pairwise correlation of <0.30 and no interaction between group and time.

3. Results

The Executive Committee stopped the trial after the second interim for pragmatic reasons related to enrollment difficulties. The decision was made without access to any by-group analyses. A total of 127 patients (licorice group n = 65, control group n = 61) were enrolled when the trial stopped, and 1 who received no trial treatment was excluded from the analysis (Figure 1).

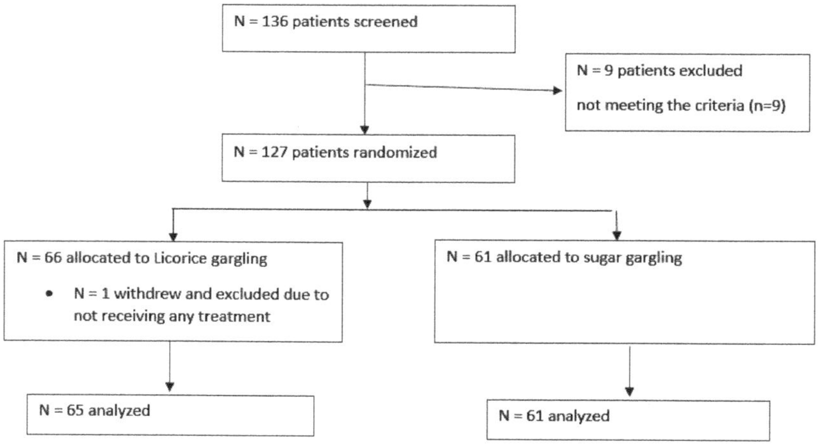

Figure 1. Patient Flowchart.

The ASA physical status and type of surgery were unbalanced and thus were adjusted for analysis. The mean ± SD ages of licorice patients was 43 ± 19 years versus 37 ± 18 years in patients randomized to sugar water (Table 1). The mean NRS results for each group within different intervals after surgery are illustrated in Table 2.

Table 2. The effect of licorice on secondary outcomes (n = 126) during PACU included 30, 60, 90, 120 min in PACU.

	Sugar (n = 61)	Licorice (n = 65)	Effect Estimate-Licorice Versus Sugar (99% CI) [b]	p Value
During PACU				
Cough incidence			Odds ratio (99.75% CI) [a]	
30 min	7 (11)	10 (15)	1.27 (0.25, 6.54)	0.656
60 min	11 (18)	3 (5)	0.19 (0.02, 1.51)	0.015
90 min	8 (13)	2 (3)	0.18 (0.02, 2.15)	0.036
120 min	6 (10)	4 (6)	0.53 (0.07, 4.16)	0.346
Until postoperative day 1 morning				
			Difference in means	
Pain score	2.8 ± 2.3	2.4 ± 2.4	−0.05 (−0.90, 0.79) [c]	0.870
			Ratio of geometric means	
Total morphine consumption, mg	14 [4, 36]	8 [4, 31]	0.93 (0.60, 1.44) [d]	0.665

Table 2. *Cont.*

	Sugar (n = 61)	Licorice (n = 65)	Effect Estimate-Licorice Versus Sugar (99% CI) [b]	p Value
POD1–POD3				
			Ratio of geometric means	
Total morphine consumption	12 [1, 25]	4 [0, 18]	0.80 (0.44, 1.47) [d]	0.346
			Difference in means	
Pain score	2.3 ± 2.2	2.3 ± 2.5	0.14 (−0.73, 1.02) [c]	0.668

Until postoperative day 1 morning included measurements in PACU and measurements afterwards until postoperative day 1 morning at 8 a.m. POD: postoperative day. Summary statistics are presented as n (%), means ± SDs, or medians [Q1, Q3]. The significance criteria was 0.01 for each secondary analysis after Bonferroni correction for multiple testing. ASA status and type of surgery were adjusted for in all the secondary analyses. (a) A generalized linear mixed model with binomial distribution with logit link assuming a covariance type of variance components (VC) to account for within-subject correlation was used. A significant treatment-by-time interaction was found on the effect of licorice on cough incidence during PACU (p = 0.080). The treatment effect was thus estimated at each separate measurement time along with 99.75% CI (0.01/4 = 0.0025) after multiple comparisons. (b) A 99% confidence interval was provided unless specified otherwise. (c) A linear mixed model assuming an autoregressive correlation structure for within subjects correlation was used to estimate the treatment effect on pain score. We did not find treatment-by-time interaction on either pain score until postoperative day 1 morning (p = 0.385) or during POD1-POD3 (p = 0.869). (d) A generalized linear model with Gaussian distribution and identity link with log transformed cumulative morphine consumption was fit to estimate the treatment effect on total morphine consumption.

We found noninferiority on pain score with an estimated difference in means of −0.09 (95.2% CI: −0.88, 0.70; p = 0.001; NI delta = 1) between licorice versus sugar gargling (Table 3). We did not find noninferiority on morphine consumption during the initial 2 postoperative hours, with an estimated ratio of geometric means of 0.85 (95.2% CI: 0.54, 1.36; p = 0.074; NI delta = 1.15) between licorice and sugar gargling. However, the absolute difference in median of morphine consumption was only 2 mg, which is not a clinically meaningful amount (Table 3). No superiority testing was conducted since we could not claim noninferiority on both primary outcomes.

Table 3. Primary noninferiority analysis: comparison on pain score and total morphine consumption during postoperative 2 h.

	Sugar (n = 61)	Licorice (n = 65)	NI Delta	Effect Estimate (95.2% CI), Noninferiority Test	Noninferiority p-Value [§]
Pain score [+]	2.9 ± 2.5	2.4 ± 2.5	1	Difference in means (Licorice versus sugar)	
				−0.09 (−0.88, 0.70)	0.001
Total morphine consumption (mg) [‡]	6 [2, 11]	4 [2, 10]	1.15	Ratio of Geometric means (Licorice versus sugar)	
				0.85 (0.54, 1.36)	0.074

NI = noninferiority; CI = confidence interval. Summary statistics are presented as means ± SDs or medians [Q1, Q3]. [§] Significant when p < 0.024 for noninferiority test in this final analysis after adjusting p value for sequential design. Noninferiority would be claimed if the upper bound of CI does not exceed the NI delta (1 for pain score and 1.15 for total morphine consumption). [+] Difference in means of pain scores were assessed using a mixed-effects model with repeated measures with an auto-regressive correlation structure. The difference on pain score was not different over time (group-by-time interaction p = 0.759). [‡] Ratio of geometric means for morphine consumption between two groups was assessed using a linear regression model after logarithm transformation on total morphine consumption.

We found a significant treatment-by-time interaction on the effect of licorice on coughing in PACU (p = 0.080). Thus, the treatment effect was estimated at each measurement time (Table 3). No significant treatment effect on coughing incidence was found at any measurement time (significance criterion = 0.0025 after multiple testing adjustment). Nor did we find any significant treatment effects for other secondary outcomes.

With the observed coefficient of variation (CV) of 0.85, we had a power of 0.18 to detect noninferiority with a noninferiority delta of 1.15 if we assume that the true ratio of geometric means is 1.0 between licorice and sugar gargling (Supplemental Figure S1) and a power of 0.78 if we assume the true ratio of geometric means is 0.8 at a significance level of 0.025 for one-sided test. The observed CV of 0.85 was higher than the 0.25 estimate used to estimate sample size, thus explaining our current actual power. Because it would have been impractical to enroll more patients, we did not conduct the planned re-estimation of the coefficient of variation.

This plot shows the power we had for detecting noninferiority on total morphine consumption with a noninferiority delta of 1.15 with different assumed treatment effects as ratios of geometric means, with observed coefficient variation of 0.85 and our current sample size of 126 at a significance level of 0.025.

4. Discussion

Previous work indicates that gargling with just 0.5 g of licorice reduces post-intubation pain and coughing [13,14]. Incisional pain is, of course, considerably more intense than post-intubation pain. We therefore used 1 g licorice dissolved in 30 g water. Nonetheless, gargling with licorice was significantly non-inferior on pain than gargling with sugar water. Morphine consumption during the initial 2 postoperative hours was not significantly non-inferior but differed by only 2 mg, which is not a clinically meaningful amount. Gargling with licorice thus provided little if any benefit on morphine consumption.

Topical analgesics and local anesthetics such as aspirin, diclofenac, ketamine, morphine, and lidocaine reportedly reduce postoperative pain, sore throat, discomfort, and even analgesic requirements within 24 h after surgery [5–12,23]. Gargling with a solution of honeysuckle and semen oroxyli (a traditional Chinese medicine) reportedly relieves both resting and swallowing throat pain during the initial 2 weeks after oropharyngeal surgery [24]. In contrast, various studies report that benzydamine hydrochloride, hydrogen peroxide oral rinses, or tantum verde mouthwash do not provide meaningful analgesia [25–27]. Two previous trials reported that gargling licorice before endotracheal intubation reduced postoperative sore throat and pain [13,14]. However, few trials directly compare the efficacy of various gargle solutions for analgesia after head and neck surgery. Our results indicate that licorice gargling provides trivial if any benefit after oropharyngeal surgery. Gargling licorice may thus reduce pain after minor airway trauma but is ineffective for more severe postsurgical pain.

Pain after head and neck surgery may partially result from colonization of bacteria in the surgical field and consequent painful inflammation—although the process presumably takes at least several hours. Oral rinses that reduce microbiological colonization and inflammation, such as hydrogen peroxide [27], benzydamine hydrochloride [26], and topical antibiotics [28], reduce postsurgical pain, presumably by reducing inflammation. A concern about perioperative licorice gargling is that the sweet herb might promote bacterial colonization within incisions, which might in turn augment pain. We saw no increase in pain over some hours, but longer-term effects remain possible. But given the lack of efficacy, it seems unlikely that licorice will be used for perioperative analgesia.

An obvious limitation of our trial is that it was stopped early for practical reasons related to low enrollment. However, there was no obvious benefit from licorice gargling, and it seems unlikely that a larger trial would demonstrate clinically meaningful benefit. Possibly a higher concentration of licorice, a different formula like gel or spray, and a combination with other anti-inflammatory and analgesic herbs would have been more effective. Sufficiently large amounts of ingested licorice can be toxic [29], but toxicity is not a concern when the herb is applied topically and not swallowed. Nonetheless, the dose is limited by the herb's intense flavor, making higher concentrations increasingly unpalatable. Another limitation is our sugar placebo. Both solutions were comparably sweet, but based on its distinctive taste, patients would surely identify licorice. Without knowing the study hypothesis, it seems unlikely that identifying licorice would provide a substantial placebo effect—especially given the observed lack of benefit.

Patients were instructed to gargle three times a day for three days, which is consistent with previous studies, which specified treatments ranging from once daily [30] to every 6 h [24]. However, we failed to assess patient compliance or evaluate the adequacy of the gargling technique once patients left the post-anesthesia care unit. Poor compliance may therefore have compromised the treatment's efficacy. Furthermore, the extent to which the intervals and duration of gargling influence analgesia remains unknown. Presumably more frequent and longer gargling would improve efficacy. It is also possible that an alternative application process would be more effective. For example, licorice lozenges would provide a longer exposure.

5. Conclusions

In summary, preinduction and postoperative licorice gargling did not produce meaningful analgesia or morphine sparing at any time during the initial three days after oropharyngeal surgery and is therefore discouraged in these patients. Our results contrast with previous trials reporting benefit from licorice gargling for less intense post-intubation sore throat. We conclude that clinicians consider alternative analgesic approaches for patients recovering from oropharyngeal surgery.

Supplementary Materials: The following supporting information can be downloaded at: https://www.mdpi.com/article/10.3390/jpm14101056/s1, Figure S1: Power to detect noninferiority on total morphine consumption in PACU assuming different treatment effect based on observed data.

Author Contributions: Conceptualization, M.W., O.P. and K.R.; methodology, M.W., M.F., O.P., D.I.S. and K.R.; validation, M.W., M.P. and K.R.; formal analysis, M.W., P.X., D.I.S. and K.R.; investigation, M.W., M.P., J.G., O.P., S.J., G.B. and W.G.; resources, M.W., O.P., D.I.S. and K.R.; data curation, M.W., P.X., D.I.S. and K.R.; writing—original draft preparation, M.W.; writing—review and editing, M.W., M.P., J.G., O.P., S.J., G.B., W.G., P.X., D.I.S. and K.R.; visualization, M.W., P.X., D.I.S. and K.R.; supervision, M.W., D.I.S. and K.R.; project administration, M.W.; funding acquisition, M.W., D.I.S. and K.R. All authors have read and agreed to the published version of the manuscript.

Funding: Departmental funding.

Institutional Review Board Statement: The study was conducted in accordance with the Declaration of Helsinki, and approved by the Institutional Review Board of Medical University of Vienna, Austria (IRB #1308/2016; 10 May 2016).

Informed Consent Statement: Informed consent was obtained from all subjects involved in the study.

Data Availability Statement: The data presented in this study are available on request from the corresponding author.

Conflicts of Interest: The authors declare no conflicts of interest.

·erences

Lee, S.; Smith, M.L.; Dahlke, D.V.; Pardo, N.; Ory, M.G. A Cross-Sectional Examination of Patients' Perspectives about Their Pain, Pain Management, and Satisfaction with Pain Treatment. *Pain Med.* **2020**, *21*, e164–e171. [CrossRef] [PubMed]

Alm, F.; Stalfors, J.; Nerfeldt, P.; Ericsson, E. Patient reported pain-related outcome measures after tonsil surgery: An analysis of 32,225 children from the National Tonsil Surgery Register in Sweden 2009-2016. *Eur. Arch. Oto-Rhino-Laryngol. Off. J. Eur. Fed. Oto-Rhino-Laryngol. Soc.* **2017**, *274*, 3711–3722. [CrossRef] [PubMed]

Eriksson, M.; Nilsson, U.; Bramhagen, A.C.; Idvall, E.; Ericsson, E. Self-reported postoperative recovery in children after tonsillectomy compared to tonsillotomy. *Int. J. Pediatr. Otorhinolaryngol.* **2017**, *96*, 47–54. [CrossRef] [PubMed]

Coulthard, P.; Haywood, D.; Tai, M.A.; Jackson-Leech, D.; Pleuvry, B.J.; Macfarlane, T.V. Treatment of postoperative pain in oral and maxillofacial surgery. *Br. J. Oral Maxillofac. Surg.* **2000**, *38*, 588–592. [CrossRef] [PubMed]

Eshghpour, M.; Mortazavi, H.; Mohammadzadeh Rezaei, N.; Nejat, A. Effectiveness of green tea mouthwash in postoperative pain control following surgical removal of impacted third molars: Double blind randomized clinical trial. *Daru J. Fac. Pharm. Tehran Univ. Med. Sci.* **2013**, *21*, 59. [CrossRef]

6. Liang, J.; Liu, J.; Qiu, Z.; Sun, G.; Xiang, P.; Hei, Z.; Li, X. Effect of Esketamine Gargle on Postoperative Sore Throat in Pati Undergoing Double-Lumen Endobronchial Intubation: A Randomised Controlled Trial. *Drug Des. Dev. Ther.* **2023**, *17*, 3139–3 [CrossRef]
7. Lisbona-Gonzalez, M.J.; Munoz-Soto, E.; Lisbona-Gonzalez, C.; Vallecillo-Rivas, M.; Diaz-Castro, J.; Moreno-Fernandez, J. Ef of Propolis Paste and Mouthwash Formulation on Healing after Teeth Extraction in Periodontal Disease. *Plants* **2021**, *10*, 1 [CrossRef]
8. Murugaiyan, A.; Sahoo, A.K.; Rao, P.B.; Misra, S. Effect of 5% EMLA Cream on Postoperative Sore Throat in Adults Follow General Endotracheal Anesthesia: A Randomized Placebo-Controlled Study. *Anesth. Analg.* **2023**, *136*, 338–345. [CrossRef]
9. Ioroi, T.; Kakei, Y.; Ito, T.; Shirai, T.; Okazaki, Y.; Hasegawa, T.; Akashi, M.; Yano, I. Efficacy and safety of ibuprofen gargle postoperative pain after mandibular third molar extraction: A phase II, placebo-controlled, double-blind, randomized crosso trial. *Clin. Exp. Dent. Res.* **2023**, *9*, 1058–1068. [CrossRef]
10. Ioroi, T.; Kiyota, N.; Imamura, Y.; Tanda, M.; Aoki, S.; Okuno, M.; Yamamoto, K.; Sasaki, R.; Nibu, K.I.; Minami, H.; e Ibuprofen gargle for chemo- or Chemoradiotherapy-induced Oral Mucositis: A feasibility study. *J. Pharm. Health Care Sci.* **2** *6*, 12. [CrossRef]
11. Mutlu, V.; Kaya, Z. Comparative efficacy of topical lidocaine, tetracaine, and articaine for post-tonsillectomy pain managemen children: A prospective, placebo-controlled study. *Acta Oto-Laryngol.* **2024**, *144*, 320–324. [CrossRef] [PubMed]
12. Puri, A.; Ghosh, S.K.; Singh, G.; Madan, A. Gargling with ketamine preoperatively decreases postoperative sore throat a endotracheal intubation in middle ear surgeries: A prospective randomized control study. *Indian J. Otolaryngol. Head Neck S Off. Publ. Assoc. Otolaryngol. India* **2022**, *74*, 5739–5743. [CrossRef] [PubMed]
13. Agarwal, A.; Gupta, D.; Yadav, G.; Goyal, P.; Singh, P.K.; Singh, U. An evaluation of the efficacy of licorice gargle for attenua postoperative sore throat: A prospective, randomized, single-blind study. *Anesth. Analg.* **2009**, *109*, 77–81. [CrossRef]
14. Ruetzler, K.; Fleck, M.; Nabecker, S.; Pinter, K.; Landskron, G.; Lassnigg, A.; You, J.; Sessler, D.I. A randomized, double-bl comparison of licorice versus sugar-water gargle for prevention of postoperative sore throat and postextubation coughing. *An Analg.* **2013**, *117*, 614–621. [CrossRef] [PubMed]
15. Batiha, G.E.; Alkazmi, L.M.; Wasef, L.G.; Beshbishy, A.M.; Nadwa, E.H.; Rashwan, E.K. Syzygium aromaticum L. (Myrtace Traditional Uses, Bioactive Chemical Constituents, Pharmacological and Toxicological Activities. *Biomolecules* **2020**, *10*, [CrossRef]
16. Dorsareh, F.; Vahid-Dastjerdi, G.; Bouyahya, A.; Zarshenas, M.M.; Rezaie, M.; Yang, W.M.; Amiri-Ardekani, E. Topical Licorice Aphthous: A Systematic Review of Clinical Trials. *Iran. J. Med. Sci.* **2023**, *48*, 437–447. [CrossRef]
17. Zhang, Y.; Yang, J.; Xie, J. Torsade de Pointes Caused by a Compound Licorice Tablet. *Int. Heart J.* **2024**, *65*, 770–774. [CrossR
18. Hautaniemi, E.J.; Tahvanainen, A.M.; Koskela, J.K.; Tikkakoski, A.J.; Kahonen, M.; Uitto, M.; Sipila, K.; Niemela, O.; Mustor J.; Porsti, I.H. Voluntary liquorice ingestion increases blood pressure via increased volume load, elevated peripheral arte resistance, and decreased aortic compliance. *Sci. Rep.* **2017**, *7*, 10947. [CrossRef]
19. Sabbadin, C.; Bordin, L.; Dona, G.; Manso, J.; Avruscio, G.; Armanini, D. Licorice: From Pseudohyperaldosteronism to Therape Uses. *Front. Endocrinol.* **2019**, *10*, 484. [CrossRef]
20. Liu, W.; Huang, S.; Li, Y.; Li, Y.; Li, D.; Wu, P.; Wang, Q.; Zheng, X.; Zhang, K. Glycyrrhizic acid from licorice down-regul inflammatory responses via blocking MAPK and PI3K/Akt-dependent NF-kappaB signalling pathways in TPA-induced s inflammation. *MedChemComm* **2018**, *9*, 1502–1510. [CrossRef]
21. Zhang, N.; Lv, H.; Shi, B.H.; Hou, X.; Xu, X. Inhibition of IL-6 and IL-8 production in LPS-stimulated human gingival fibrobl by glycyrrhizin via activating LXRalpha. *Microb. Pathog.* **2017**, *110*, 135–139. [CrossRef] [PubMed]
22. Honarmand, A.; Safavi, M.; Safaei Arani, A.; Shokrani, O. The efficacy of different doses of liquorice gargling for attenuat postoperative sore throat and cough after tracheal intubation. *Eur. J. Anaesthesiol.* **2016**, *33*, 595–596. [CrossRef]
23. Nielsen, B.N.; Friis, S.M.; Schmiegelow, K.; Henneberg, S.; Romsing, J. Evaluation of topical morphine for treatment of mucositis in cancer patients. *Br. J. Pain* **2021**, *15*, 411–419. [CrossRef]
24. Ren, L.; Li, J.; Miao, Z.; Yan, R.; Li, Q.; Zhang, R.; Rong, T.; Dong, X. The application of gargle containing honeysuckle and sen oroxyli to reduce the pain and complications after uvulopalatopharyngoplasty. *Front. Pharmacol.* **2022**, *13*, 974233. [CrossRe
25. Goswami, D.; Jain, G.; Mohod, M.; Baidya, D.K.; Bhutia, O.; Roychoudhury, A. Randomized controlled trial to comp oral analgesic requirements and patient satisfaction in using oral non-steroidal anti-inflammatory drugs versus benzydan hydrochloride oral rinses after mandibular third molar extraction: A pilot study. *J. Dent. Anesth. Pain Med.* **2018**, *18*, 19- [CrossRef] [PubMed]
26. Hanani, T.; Gadban, H.; Jahshan, F.; Ronen, O. Tantum verde mouthwash for tonsillectomy: A prospective, double-bl randomized control trial. *Int. J. Pediatr. Otorhinolaryngol.* **2019**, *121*, 173–178. [CrossRef] [PubMed]
27. Chacra, Z.A.; Manoukian, J.J.; Al-Qahtani, K.; Al-Eisa, M.; Balys, R.; Hagr, A.; Tewfik, T.L.; Schloss, M.D. Hydrogen pero mouth rinse: An analgesic post-tonsillectomy. *J. Otolaryngol.* **2005**, *34*, 178–182. [CrossRef]
28. Cho, H.; Lynham, A.J.; Hsu, E. Postoperative interventions to reduce inflammatory complications after third molar surg Review of the current evidence. *Aust. Dent. J.* **2017**, *62*, 412–419. [CrossRef]

Nazari, S.; Rameshrad, M.; Hosseinzadeh, H. Toxicological Effects of Glycyrrhiza glabra (Licorice): A Review. *Phytother. Res. PTR* **2017**, *31*, 1635–1650. [CrossRef]
Kakei, Y.; Ioroi, T.; Ito, T.; Okazaki, Y.; Hasegawa, T.; Yano, I.; Akashi, M. Efficacy of Ibuprofen Gargle for Postoperative Pain After Mandibular Third Molar Extraction: Protocol for a Phase II, Placebo-Controlled, Double-Blind, Randomized Crossover Trial. *JMIR Res. Protoc.* **2022**, *11*, e35533. [CrossRef]

Journal of
Personalized Medicine

MD

Systematic Review

Endoscopic Sinus Surgery in Frontal Sinus Inverted Papilloma: A Systematic Review

Maxime Fieux [1,2,*], Valentin Favier [3,4], Andre Sousa Machado [5,6], Mikail Nourredine [7], Caroline Giroudon [8], Florent Carsuzaa [9,10], Paresh P. Naik [11] and the yo-IFOS Group

1 Hospices Civils de Lyon, Centre Hospitalier Lyon Sud, Service d'ORL, d'Otoneurochirurgie et de Chirurgie Cervico-Faciale, 69495 Pierre Bénite, France
2 Université de Lyon, Université Lyon 1, 69003 Lyon, France
3 Département d'ORL, Chirurgie Cervico Faciale et Maxillo-Faciale, Hôpital Gui de Chauliac, CHU de Montpellier, 34295 Montpellier, France; valentin_favier@hotmail.com
4 Research-Team ICAR, Laboratory of Computer Science, Robotics and Microelectronics of Montpellier (LIRMM), Université de Montpellier, French National Centre for Scientific Research (CNRS), 34095 Montpellier, France
5 Department of Otolaryngology, Unidade Local de Saúde de Trás-os-Montes e Alto (ULSTMAD), CP 5000-508 Vila Real, Portugal; sousamachado.andre@gmail.com
6 Faculty of Health Sciences, University of Beira Interior, CP 6200-506 Covilhã, Portugal
7 Service de Biostatistiques de Lyon, Pôle Santé Publique, Hospices Civil de Lyon, 69002 Lyon, France; mikail.nourredine@chu-lyon.fr
8 Service de la Documentation Centrale, Hospices Civils de Lyon, 69424 Lyon, France; caroline.giroudon@chu-lyon.fr
9 Service ORL, Chirurgie Cervico-Maxillo-Faciale et Audiophonologie, Centre Hospitalier Universitaire de Poitiers, 86000 Poitiers, France; florent.carsuzaa@gmail.com
10 Laboratoire Inflammation Tissus Epithéliaux et Cytokines (LITEC), UR15560, Université de Poitiers, 86000 Poitiers, France
11 Jaslok Hospital & Research Centre, Pedder Road, Mumbai, Maharashtra 400026, India; pareshnaikp@gmail.com
* Correspondence: maxime.fieux@chu-lyon.fr

Abstract: Background: Frontal sinus inverted papilloma (IP) is a particularly rare form of IP and its management is challenging, with a high rate of recurrence. **Objectives**: Our aim was to evaluate the recurrence rate of frontal sinus IP after surgery and compare this rate according to the surgical modality (purely endoscopic sinus surgery vs. a combined/open approach). **Design**: A systematic review without meta-analysis conducted by a working group of the Young Otolaryngologists of the International Federation of Otorhinolaryngological Societies (yo-IFOS). **Data Sources and Methods**: A systematic analysis of the literature was performed and reported following the criteria laid down in the SWiM guidelines. The review was registered on Prospero, a dedicated software was used for screening (Covidence), and R (v.4.2.2) was used for statistical analysis. Eligible articles were studies reporting at least five cases of frontal sinus IP surgically treated. **Results**: A total of 2925 studies were identified based on the MeSH equation, and 39 studies were included (n = 642 patients). Among the studies included, the recurrence rate was 18.4% (118/642) with a mean time to recurrence of 25.6 (±11.7) months. The difference between surgical modalities was not statistically significant in terms of recurrence rate (14.7% vs. 16.5%; $p = 0.675$). **Conclusions**: The recurrence rate of frontal sinus IP is not different between surgical modalities. However, it does not reduce the need for a tailored therapeutic strategy, as other factors also need to be considered (time to recurrence, complications, quality of life) when choosing the most appropriate approach.

Keywords: sinus surgery; endoscopic sinus surgery; inverted papilloma; frontal sinus; recurrence

1. Introduction

Sinonasal inverted papilloma (IP) is a rare benign neoplasm accounting for 0.5–4% of nasal sinus neoplasms [1,2]. There is a male predominance, a male-to-female ratio of 3.4:1, and a mean age of 55 years [3], and an incidence of 0.01 to 0.33/100,000 person–years [4]. Although smoking, viral infections, diabetes, allergies, and chronic inflammation are possible causes, human papillomavirus (HPV) is considered a significant cofactor in the pathogenesis—especially types 6, 11, 16, and 18 [5,6]. Recent reports have also suggested that occupational exposure is a risk factor for sinonasal IP [7]. Sinonasal IP has a recurrence rate of 15–30%, with locally aggressive features that lead to the destruction of adjacent bony structures and the compression of neurovascular adjacent structures. Recurrence is defined here as any positive imaging or endoscopic abnormalities where biopsies were performed and recurrence histologically proven. It is also known that IP is associated with malignant transformation, with a rate of transformation into squamous cell carcinoma (SCC) between 7 and 9% [3,8]. As a result, an extended surgical excision is essential, requiring the removal and drilling of the tumor's bony attachment point [9]. Sinonasal IP treatment has evolved from an open surgery to a purely endoscopic sinus surgery. The most frequent site of attachment is the lateral nasal wall, followed by the maxillary and ethmoid sinuses and walls. Less commonly, IP can arise in the frontal sinus, nasal septum, or sphenoid sinus [10,11]. The size and origin of the tumor can be preoperatively determined using imaging with an accuracy of 74–90%. They are both of the utmost importance for surgical planning and success [10].

Frontal sinus IP is a particularly rare form of this condition, representing only 2.5–5% of all IP cases [12,13]. Frontal sinus IP is suspected to carry a higher likelihood of recurrence compared to IP arising in other areas of the sinonasal cavity [12,14]. However, there is currently no robust data in the literature to support this point. Indeed, most authors use the Krouse classification [15], which gathers the frontal, sphenoid, and non-medial maxillary wall locations in stage III. When feasible, a purely endoscopic sinus surgery is the preferred treatment method for frontal sinus IP. This is due to its favorable outcomes and lower morbidity compared to more invasive open surgery [16]. Some challenging anatomical factors, such as limited access to the tumor's pedicle, may dictate a combined surgical approach (endoscopic and open approach). This kind of combined approach enables its total removal and regional control [11].

The aim of this systematic review, conducted by a working group of the Young Otolaryngologists of the International Federation of Otorhinolaryngological Societies (YO-IFOS), was to evaluate the recurrence rate of frontal sinus IP after surgery and compare this rate according to the surgical modality (purely endoscopic sinus surgery or combined/open approach).

2. Materials and Methods

2.1. Synthesis Without Meta-Analysis Criteria

The systematic analysis of the literature was performed and reported following the criteria laid down in the Synthesis Without Meta-Analysis guidelines (SWiM) [17] and the PRISMA checklist (attached) to ensure that the research strategy and statistics would be reproductible.

2.2. Protocol and Registration

The study was registered in the Prospero database in April 2024 (n° CRD42023487678) as a systematic review of health research studies including human subjects.

2.3. Inclusion Criteria

Eligible articles were articles reporting original clinical or preclinical research on modalities, effectiveness, and the safety of surgical treatment of frontal sinus IP, published in the medical literature at any time between 1960 and 2024. Although the inclusion period began in 1960, we performed a sensitivity analysis focused on studies published after 2000 to assess consistency with modern surgical techniques. Only articles reporting the main outcome (i.e., the exact number of recurrences from IP emerging from the frontal sinus) were included. The human studies included randomized controlled trials (RCTs), non-randomized controlled trials, and observational studies. Systematic analyses, with or without meta-analyses, narrative analyses, and case reports of a single patient were excluded. Reviews, although not included, were examined individually to analyze their reference lists for articles liable to meet the inclusion criteria.

2.4. Sources

Studies were identified in the Pubmed/Medline (US National Library of Medicine), Web of Science (Clarivate), CENTRAL, SciELO and Embase (Elsevier) databases. They were queried on 04/24/2024. Further references were sought in the articles' reference lists. Automatic alerts were set up for each database to monitor the publication of studies likely to enrich the work during the writing and analysis phase. The literature watch was continued up to 15 March 2025 (submission).

2.5. Literature Search Strategy

The search formula was drawn up using Medical Subject Headings (MeSH) and free-text abbreviations and terms relating to allergic and non-allergic rhinitis. Keywords included but were not limited to "Papilloma, Inverted" AND "Frontal Sinus" OR "Paranasal Sinus Neoplasms" OR "Paranasal Sinuses". We did not use a time limit in our research. Only studies published in the following languages were selected: English, French, Spanish, Italian, German, and Portuguese. The search formulae were defined by an information specialist of the Lyon university hospitals (C.G.); the MeSH and free-text equations are detailed in the Supplementary Material S1.

2.6. Article Selection

Figure 1 shows the SWiM flowchart for article selection drawn up using Covidence, which was used to carry out the double-blind screening work. Retrieved citations and abstracts were compiled in a single reference list. The software eliminated duplicates. Selection proceeded in two phases: the selection of titles and abstracts (MF, PN), then selection on full text (VF, ASM). Relevant articles were examined in greater depth, and those not meeting the inclusion criteria were rejected. In case of disagreement, a third opinion was sought from another investigator (FC). If the data in the abstract were insufficient for a decision, the full text of the article was obtained and read. When full text was not available (presentations or lectures), an inter-library loan was requested and, if the full text was still not available, the article was excluded. The full-text articles included were examined to extract title, author, date, journal, number of references, type of study, surgical modality, sample size, gender, age, follow-up duration, type of intervention, Krouse classification, recurrence rate, time to recurrence, complications, and risk of bias; these data were entered in a standardized Microsoft Excel® spreadsheet for systematic reviews.

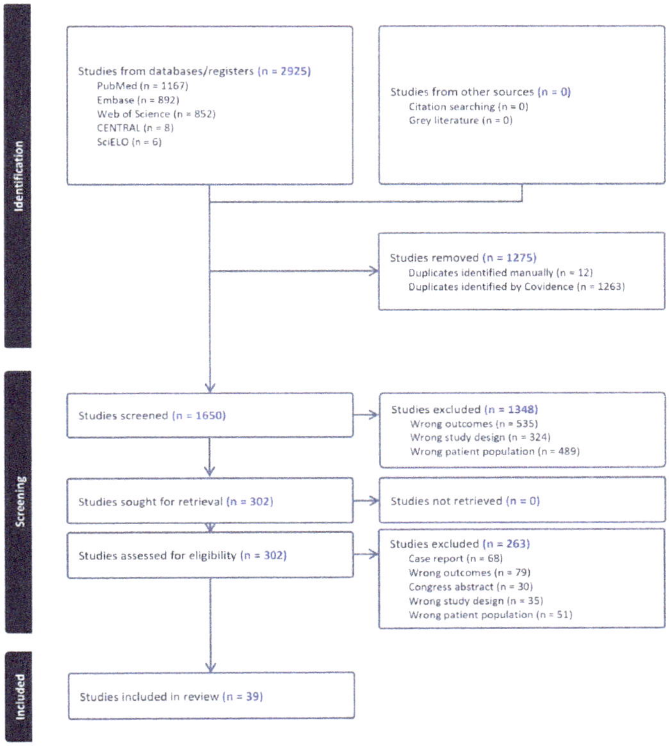

Figure 1. SWiM flowchart. Footnotes: The flowchart was automatically generated using the software Covidence, which enabled double-blind screening for both phases (title and abstract; full text).

2.7. Data Collection and Selection

Data were extracted from texts, tables, or graphs. International units were used, with conversion as necessary. Continuous data were used if possible, and dichotomous or categoric variables if not.

2.8. Risk of Bias Assessment Methods

The bias analysis was carried out by two investigators (MF, VF) using the Methodological Index for Non-Randomized Studies (MINORS) tool, which is a validated instrument designed for assessing the quality of non-randomized surgical studies [18]. The MINORS tool consists of 12 items related to the analysis of methodological points of comparative (ideal score = 24) and non-comparative studies (ideal score = 16).

2.9. Main Results

The main outcome was the proportion of recurrence after surgery in patients with frontal sinus IP. The secondary outcome was the comparison of recurrence rate according to the surgical modality, i.e., purely endoscopic sinus surgery or other surgical approach. The latter was defined herein as either open surgery alone or open and endoscopic surgery combined. First, the demographics, surgical modalities, type of intervention (primary or revision surgery), quality of life scores, safety (minor and major adverse events), and tumor characteristics (Krouse classification) of the included studies were described. A minimum of 5 studies was considered sufficient to perform such a descriptive analysis. Then, the main and secondary outcomes were reported. Finally, the risk of bias was assessed. Data analysis was performed using R software (version 4.3.3).

3. Results

3.1. Study Selection

A total of 2925 studies were identified based on the MeSH equation; 302 were assessed for full-text screening after duplicates (n = 1275) and non-eligible studies based on the title and abstract were excluded (n = 1348, Figure 1). Finally, 39 studies (n = 642 patients), all observational, were included in the analysis—34 of these met the initial inclusion criteria and 5 were added based on the literature update pursued until submission. The majority of included studies (97.4%) were published after 2000 (only 1 was published in 1995).

3.2. Description of Included Studies

Among the 39 studies included [12,14,16,19–54], 16 (±14) patients per study were included in average, at a mean age of 55.5 (±3.5) years old, and for a mean follow-up of 39.8 (±17.9) months. There was a male-to-female ratio favoring males, with 70.4% male patients (152/216; data available for 6 studies) [16,22,41,47,49,51]. Regarding surgical modality, data were available for 64.0% of studies (25/39; n = 485 patients); a total of 71.3% (346/485) of patients underwent purely endoscopic sinus surgery and the other 28.7% (139/485) underwent other approaches (Table 1). Type of intervention (primary or revision surgery), quality of life, safety, and Krouse classification could not be included in the analysis because of a lack of data regarding the specific frontal sinus location (less than 5 studies had available data).

Table 1. Comparison between surgical modalities.

Characteristics (n = 25 Studies)	Other Approaches	Purely Endoscopic	*p*-Value
Mean number of patients per study (±SD)	5.6 (7.0)	13.8 (15.2)	0.003
Age in years (±SD)	59.0 (5.6)	52.6 (2.8)	0.095
Follow-up in months (±SD)	40.2 (0.4)	30.7 (11.7)	0.381
Rate of recurrence	16.5%	14.7%	0.675
Time to recurrence; n = 5 studies	73.2 (40.8)	28.0 (11.3)	0.095

Numeric variables were expressed as mean with standard deviations (SD) and discrete outcomes as absolute and relative (%) frequencies. Other approaches were either open surgery alone or open and endoscopic surgery combined.

3.3. Recurrence Rate After Surgery in Frontal Sinus IP

Among the 39 studies included, the recurrence rate was 18.4% (118/642) with a mean time to recurrence of 25.6 (±11.7) months. Among patients who underwent purely endoscopic sinus surgery, the recurrence rate was 14.7% (51/346) compared to 16.5% (23/139) in patients who underwent other approaches (p = 0.675). Regarding time to recurrence, which was available in five studies [19,20,30,39,49], it was 28.0 (±11.3) months in patients who underwent a purely endoscopic sinus surgery and 73.2 (±40.8) months in patients who underwent other approaches with no significant difference (p = 0.095; Table 1).

3.4. Risk of Bias Assessment

Among the 39 studies included, 25 had a control group and were considered as comparative studies. The mean MINORS score for all studies included was 13.1 (±2.8). Among the comparative studies (n = 25), the mean MINORS score was 15.1/24 (±0.99), and among the non-comparative ones (n = 14), the mean MINORS score was 9.6/16 (±0.93; Table 2).

Table 2. Synthesis of included studies.

Author. Year	Sample Size (n)	Age (Years)	Follow up (Month)	Recurrence (n)	Recurrence Time (Month)	MINOR Score	MINOR Maximum Score
Lawson. 1995 [35]	7	57.3	54.0	3	NA	11	16
Bertrand. 2000 [22]	85	58.4	41.9	15	8	16	24
Lawson. 2003 [36]	13	NA	NA	3	NA	14	24
Dubin. 2005 [27]	6	NA	NA	5	13.3	14	24
on Buchwald. 2005 [48]	13	61.0	37.0	0	9	16	24
Minovi. 2006 [39]	13	NA	NA	0	NA	14	24
Holzmann. 2007 [31]	9	NA	35.0	1	35	11	16
Woodworth. 2007 [53]	9	NA	40	4	NA	11	16
Sautter. 2007 [43]	5	55.0	NA	0	16.8	14	24
Kim. 2008 [34]	5	51.4	41.9	0	NA	16	24
Zhang. 2008 [51]	9	50.2	15.1	0	NA	15	24
Yoon. 2009 [49]	18	55.0	36.6	4	36	16	24
Dragonetti. 2011 [26]	8	NA	NA	1	NA	14	24
Lombardi. 2011 [37]	27	NA	NA	2	NA	14	24
Kamel. 2012 [32]	6	49.0	27.0	0	NA	16	24
Kim. 2012 [14]	22	54.1	41.0	6	32.6	16	24
Sciarretta. 2014 [44]	9	58.7	18.0	2	18	14	24
Promsopa. 2015 [42]	17	55.0	7.5	0	7.5	10	16
Adriaensen. 2015 [20]	20	53.7	47.6	2	42	16	24
Karligkiotis. 2015 [33]	5	48.0	40.6	0	NA	16	24
Akkari. 2016 [21]	12	NA	NA	3	23.6	9	16
Nygren. 2016 [40]	10	NA	NA	10	NA	9	16
Takahashi. 2016 [46]	10	58.4	39.5	0	NA	11	16
Adriaensen. 2016 [19]	17	NA	NA	3	26.6	14	24
Healy. 2016 [30]	26	56.9	96.0	4	32.4	16	24
Verillaud. 2016 [47]	27	58.0	40.0	2	40	16	24
Choi. 2019 [24]	23	NA	NA	6	37.76	9	16
Pietrobon. 2019 [41]	47	57.0	43.0	2	24	16	24
Coutinho. 2020 [25]	5	NA	NA	1	11.4	9	16
Ferrari. 2020 [28]	12	NA	NA	1	34	9	16
Lee. 2020 [12]	14	NA	NA	9	NA	14	24
Sham. 2020 [45]	29	55.0	56.4	12	39.8	16	24
Minni. 2021 [38]	21	NA	NA	3	NA	14	24
Glikson. 2022 [29]	17	NA	NA	3	NA	9	16
Yu. 2023 [50]	9	NA	NA	1	NA	14	24
Cho. 2024 [23]	13	60.6	NA	0	NA	9	16
Delaine. 2024 [52]	5	55.5	NA	3	23.8	9	16
mimiArdestani. 2024 [54]	9	NA	NA	4	NA	9	16
Gaudioso. 2024 [16]	30	57	37	3	NA	16	24

For each study, first author, date of publication, sample size (number of patients per study), recurrence details, and MINORS score is given. NA; not available.

4. Discussion

This systematic review included 39 studies corresponding to 642 patients, representing one of the largest systematic reviews to date with a focus on frontal sinus IP. The overall recurrence rate was 18.4%, and although it was not statistically different, the recurrence rate appeared to be lower among patients who underwent a purely endoscopic sinus surgery (14.7%) compared to those with other approaches (16.5%).

The demographics of the population suffering from frontal sinus IP described herein was similar to that of patients with IP of other locations, with a mean age of 55 years at diagnosis, as described in other locations (maxillary, ethmoid, or others), and a difference in male-to-female ratio [3,4,12]. However, the latter might be subject to sampling bias, as data were missing for 33 studies and should thus be considered with caution.

In the present study, the mean follow-up was 40 months with a recurrence rate of 14.7% for the purely endoscopic sinus surgery group, which is comparable to the described recurrence rate of 15% after endoscopic resection for IP of other locations [55]. The results herein are concordant with the literature. In a recent review of the literature on the long-term follow-up of IP, Kuan et al. found a recurrence rate of 16.1% (±9.1%) with a mean time to recurrence ranging from 8 to 45.5 months [11]. One of the hypotheses supporting this result is the role of endoscope magnification, which helps to clean the surgical field as easily as during an open approach in carefully selected patients [56].

In the present study, the mean recurrence rate of frontal sinus IP was 18.7% (121/647) with no significant difference found between purely endoscopic and combined approaches. Similarly, Gaudioso et al. recently reviewed the surgical outcomes of frontal IP [16]. They included both frontal sinus and frontal recess locations of the pedicle and found a similar 18.9% rate of recurrence. However, they found a higher recurrence rate when combined approaches were performed without osteoplastic flaps (not studied herein). This difference could be explained by how the authors grouped frontal sinus IP. Authors believe that given the widespread use of endoscopic sinus surgery even for extended approaches, purely intra-frontal and frontal recess IP should be distinguished, as the second one is not so difficult to access. Further data are needed as, to date, the difference is not clear within the available literature.

In most studies, the mode of frontal sinus involvement (i.e., bulging tumor or tumor pedicle) was not reported. Kim et al. found 17 cases of frontal sinus IP in a Korean multicenter study involving 939 patients, and among them, the frontal sinus was the origin site in 3% of cases, but the frontal sinus was involved in 16.6% of cases [14]. A more precise description of the IP implantation site should be performed to allow for a comparison between open/combined and purely endoscopic approaches for future studies. This description could be based on already existing classifications, such as the one on malignant tumors proposed by Bastier et al. [57]. The latter enables a precise description of the pedicle location. This detail is the most important factor in preventing the recurrence, as described by Adriaensen et al. [19]. Also, the completeness of resection in the primary endoscopic surgery is of course essential and should remain the main goal for every patient. The authors believe that the Krouse classification [15] is not up to date anymore, which is necessary to ensure a precise description of the origin site of the tumor in frontal sinus IP, and it could be one of the future aims of the European Position Paper on Sinus (EPOS).

Furthermore, several methodological limitations affect the strength of the evidence. There was no double-blind randomized controlled trials, and among the included studies, the number of studies with details regarding the surgical modalities were low. Due to inconsistent reporting of tumor staging, particularly the Krouse classification, we were unable to assess the potential impact of tumor stage on recurrence. This constitutes a major limitation in interpreting surgical outcomes. Overall, most of the studies analyzed had a high risk of bias. This risk is attributed to study designs and precisions on the surgical modalities and tumor location, which directly limits the strength and generalizability of our conclusions.

The authors wish to highlight that they conducted a comprehensive and rigorous search of literature on frontal sinus IP, which ultimately yielded 39 studies. However, the heterogeneity among these studies was high, both in methodology and in reporting, which inherently limits the strength of the conclusions one could draw. This is a recognized challenge in systematic reviews on rare and complex pathologies such as frontal sinus IP. The authors intentionally focused their analysis on endpoints that were consistently and explicitly reported across studies—namely, the surgical approach and recurrence rate. While many additional factors can influence recurrence, such as tumor extent, surgeon experience, and follow-up duration, the available data did not allow for a detailed subgroup analysis of these variables. Nonetheless, recurrence remains a clinically relevant endpoint that strongly influences surgical decision making, and we believe that synthesizing the currently available data provides value to the field. This clarification underscores our cautious interpretation of the findings and the incremental contribution of this systematic review to the ongoing discussion on optimal management strategies for frontal sinus IP. Different factors should be mentioned when performing a study on frontal sinus IP. Among them, the preoperative suspected location of the IP pedicle [58], the preoperative risk of malignant transformation [59], the reasons to choose an either purely endoscopic or combined approach (imaging data, tumor characteristics, and the experience of the surgeon), and the final location of the pedicle during the surgery are particularly important factors. Although, pre-operative informed consent from the patient is mandatory and it should be mentioned that even in case of an endoscopic approach, a possible conversion into an open approach might be needed [60].

5. Conclusions

Even if no robust conclusion could be drawn, it seems that the recurrence rate of frontal sinus IP is not different between surgical modalities. However, it does not reduce the need for a tailored therapeutic strategy, as other factors also need to be considered (time to recurrence, complications, quality of life) when choosing the most appropriate approach.

Supplementary Materials: The following supporting information can be downloaded at: https://www.mdpi.com/article/10.3390/jpm15050183/s1, Supplementary Materials S1: MeSH equations.

Author Contributions: All authors contributed to the study conception and design as well as the drafting of the article. M.F. was responsible for the statistical analysis of the data. P.P.N., A.S.M., V.F. and F.C. revised the study critically for important intellectual content, and all authors gave final approval of the version to be submitted. All authors have read and agreed to the published version of the manuscript.

Funding: This research received no external funding.

Institutional Review Board Statement: Not Applicable.

Informed Consent Statement: Not applicable.

Data Availability Statement: Original data are available on request.

Acknowledgments: We thank Véréna Landel (Direction de le Recherche en Santé, Hospices Civils de Lyon) for her help in manuscript preparation. M.F. is supported by the Foundation of the Hospices Civil de Lyon fellowship and wishes to acknowledge the support of the Fondation Edmond

Roudnitska (two grants awarded), the Philippe Foundation (grant awarded), the France-Stanford Centre (grant awarded).

Conflicts of Interest: The authors declare no conflicts of interest.

Abbreviations

The following abbreviations are used in this manuscript:

IP	Inverted Papilloma
MINORS	Methodological Index for Non-Randomized Studies
SWIM	Systematic Review without Meta-Analysis
EPOS	European Position Paper on Sinus

References

1. Wang, M.; Noel, J.E. Etiology of Sinonasal Inverted Papilloma: A Narrative Review. *World J. Otorhinolaryngol.-Head Neck S* **2017**, *3*, 54–58. [CrossRef] [PubMed]
2. Vorasubin, N.; Vira, D.; Suh, J.D.; Bhuta, S.; Wang, M.B. Schneiderian Papillomas: Comparative Review of Exophytic, Oncoc and Inverted Types. *Am. J. Rhinol. Allergy* **2013**, *27*, 287–292. [CrossRef]
3. Lisan, Q.; Laccourreye, O.; Bonfils, P. Sinonasal Inverted Papilloma: From Diagnosis to Treatment. *Eur. Ann. Otorhinolary Head Neck Dis.* **2016**, *133*, 337–341. [CrossRef] [PubMed]
4. Elliot, A.; Marklund, L.; Håkansson, N.; Song, H.; Ye, W.; Stjärne, P.; Hammarstedt-Nordenvall, L. Incidence of IP and Ris Malignant Transformation in the Swedish Population 1960–2010. *Eur. Arch. Oto-Rhino-Laryngol.* **2017**, *274*, 1445–1448. [Cross [PubMed]
5. Lawson, W.; Schlecht, N.F.; Brandwein-Gensler, M. The Role of the Human Papillomavirus in the Pathogenesis of Schneide Inverted Papillomas: An Analytic Overview of the Evidence. *Head Neck Pathol.* **2008**, *2*, 49–59. [CrossRef]
6. Govindaraj, S.; Wang, H. Does Human Papilloma Virus Play a Role in Sinonasal Inverted Papilloma? *Curr. Opin. Otolary Head Neck Surg.* **2014**, *22*, 47–51. [CrossRef]
7. d'Errico, A.; Zajacova, J.; Cacciatore, A.; Baratti, A.; Zanelli, R.; Alfonzo, S.; Beatrice, F. Occupational Risk Factors for Sinon Inverted Papilloma: A Case–Control Study. *Occup. Environ. Med.* **2013**, *70*, 703–708. [CrossRef]
8. Buchwald, C.; Franzmann, M.; Tos, M. Sinonasal Papillomas: A Report of 82 Cases in Copenhagen County, Includi Longitudinal Epidemiological and Clinical Study. *Laryngoscope* **1995**, *105*, 72–79. [CrossRef]
9. Kamel, R.H.; Khaled, A.; Abdelfattah, A.F.; Awad, A.G. Surgical Treatment of Sinonasal Inverted Papilloma. *Curr. O Otolaryngol. Head Neck Surg.* **2022**, *30*, 26–32. [CrossRef]
10. Russo, C.; Elefante, A.; Romano, A.; Cama, A.; Erra, M.; Ugga, L.; Brunetti, L.; Motta, G.; Califano, L.; Iengo, M.; et al Multimodal Diagnostic Approach to Inverted Papilloma: Proposal of a Novel Diagnostic Flow-Chart. *Curr. Probl. Diagn. Ra* **2021**, *50*, 499–504. [CrossRef]
11. Kuan, E.C.; Wang, E.W.; Adappa, N.D.; Beswick, D.M.; London, N.R.; Su, S.Y.; Wang, M.B.; Abuzeid, W.M.; Alexiev, B.; J.A.; et al. International Consensus Statement on Allergy and Rhinology: Sinonasal Tumors. *Int. Forum Allergy Rhinol.* **2024** 149–608. [CrossRef] [PubMed]
12. Lee, J.J.; Roland, L.T.; Licata, J.J.; Orlowski, H.L.P.; Jiramongkolchai, P.; Piccirillo, J.F.; Kallogjeri, D.; Klatt-Cromwell, C Chernock, R.D.; Schneider, J.S. Morphologic, Intraoperative, and Histologic Risk Factors for Sinonasal Inverted Papill Recurrence. *Laryngoscope* **2020**, *130*, 590–596. [CrossRef] [PubMed]
13. Shohet, J.; Duncavage, J. Management of the Frontal Sinus with Inverted Papilloma. *Otolaryngol. Head Neck Surg.* **1996**, 649–652. [CrossRef] [PubMed]
14. Kim, D.-Y.; Hong, S.-L.; Lee, C.H.; Jin, H.-R.; Kang, J.M.; Lee, B.-J.; Moon, I.J.; Chung, S.-K.; Rha, K.-S.; Cho, S.H.; et al. Inver Papilloma of the Nasal Cavity and Paranasal Sinuses: A Korean Multicenter Study. *Laryngoscope* **2012**, *122*, 487–494. [CrossR
15. Krouse, J.H. Development of a Staging System for Inverted Papilloma. *Laryngoscope* **2000**, *110*, 965–968. [CrossRef]
16. Gaudioso, P.; Vinciguerra, A.; Verillaud, B.; Herman, P. Management of Frontal Sinus and Frontal Recess Inverted Papilloma: Experience and Systematic Review. *Acta Otorhinolaryngol. Ital.* **2024**, *44*, 252–260. [CrossRef]
17. Campbell, M.; McKenzie, J.E.; Sowden, A.; Katikireddi, S.V.; Brennan, S.E.; Ellis, S.; Hartmann-Boyce, J.; Ryan, R.; Shepperd Thomas, J.; et al. Synthesis without Meta-Analysis (SWiM) in Systematic Reviews: Reporting Guideline. *BMJ* **2020**, *368*, l6 [CrossRef]

Slim, K.; Nini, E.; Forestier, D.; Kwiatkowski, F.; Panis, Y.; Chipponi, J. Methodological Index for Non-Randomized Studies (Minors): Development and Validation of a New Instrument. *ANZ J. Surg.* **2003**, *73*, 712–716. [CrossRef]
Adriaensen, G.F.J.P.M.; Lim, K.-H.; Georgalas, C.; Reinartz, S.M.; Fokkens, W.J. Challenges in the Management of Inverted Papilloma: A Review of 72 Revision Cases. *Laryngoscope* **2016**, *126*, 322–328. [CrossRef]
Adriaensen, G.F.; van der Hout, M.W.; Reinartz, S.M.; Georgalas, C.; Fokkens, W.J. Endoscopic Treatment of Inverted Papilloma Attached in the Frontal Sinus/Recess. *Rhinology* **2015**, *53*, 317–324. [CrossRef]
Akkari, M.; Lassave, J.; Mura, T.; Gascou, G.; Pierre, G.; Cartier, C.; Garrel, R.; Crampette, L. Atypical Presentations of Sinonasal Inverted Papilloma: Surgical Management and Influence on the Recurrence Rate. *Am. J. Rhinol. Allergy* **2016**, *30*, 149–154. [CrossRef]
Bertrand, B.; Eloy, P.; Jorissen, M.; Rombaux, P.; Daele, J.; Boniver, V.; Collet, S.; Demanez, J.P.; Verheyden, P.J.; Bachert, C. Surgery of Inverted Papillomas under Endoscopic Control. *Acta Otorhinolaryngol. Belg.* **2000**, *54*, 139–150. [PubMed]
Cho, S.W.; Kim, S.G.; Han, D.H.; Kim, H.J.; Kim, J.W.; Kim, D.Y.; Rhee, C.S.; Won, T.B. Treatment Outcome and Prognostic Factors of Inverted Papilloma Involving the Frontal Sinus. *Laryngoscope Investig. Otolaryngol.* **2024**, *9*, e1206. [CrossRef] [PubMed]
Choi, W.R.; Lee, B.J.; Kim, J.H. Long-Term Outcome Following Resection of Sinonasal Inverted Papillomas: A Single Surgeon's Experience in 127 Patients. *Clin. Otolaryngol.* **2019**, *44*, 652–655. [CrossRef]
Coutinho, G.; Marques, J.; Leal, M.; Spratley, J.; Fernandes, M.S.; Santos, M. Surgical Outcomes of Sinonasal Inverted Papilloma: A 17 Year Review. *Braz. J. Otorhinolaryngol.* **2020**, *86*, 315–320. [CrossRef]
Dragonetti, A.; Gera, R.; Sciuto, A.; Scotti, A.; Bigoni, A.; Barbaro, E.; Minni, A. Sinonasal Inverted Papilloma: 84 Patients Treated by Endoscopy and Proposal for a New Classification. *Rhinology* **2011**, *49*, 207–213. [CrossRef]
Dubin, M.G.; Sonnenburg, R.E.; Melroy, C.T.; Ebert, C.S.; Coffey, C.S.; Senior, B.A. Staged Endoscopic and Combined Open/Endoscopic Approach in the Management of Inverted Papilloma of the Frontal Sinus. *Am. J. Rhinol.* **2005**, *19*, 442–445. [CrossRef] [PubMed]
Ferrari, M.; Schreiber, A.; Mattavelli, D.; Rampinelli, V.; Bertazzoni, G.; Tomasoni, M.; Gualtieri, T.; Nicolai, P. How Aggressive Should Resection of Inverted Papilloma Be? Refinement of Surgical Planning Based on the 25-Year Experience of a Single Tertiary Center. *Int. Forum. Allergy Rhinol.* **2020**, *10*, 619–628. [CrossRef]
Glikson, E.; Dragonetti, A.; Soudry, E.; Rozendoren, N.; Alon, E.E.; Landsberg, R.; Schneider, S.; Bedrin, L.; Mozzanica, F.; Bulgheroni, C.; et al. Is Intraoperative Margin Sampling Necessary in Inverted Papilloma Resection? *Eur. Arch. Otorhinolaryngol.* **2022**, *279*, 2935–2942. [CrossRef]
Healy, D.Y., Jr.; Chhabra, N.; Metson, R.; Holbrook, E.H.; Gray, S.T. Surgical Risk Factors for Recurrence of Inverted Papilloma. *Laryngoscope* **2016**, *126*, 796–801. [CrossRef]
Holzmann, D.; Hegyi, I.; Rajan, G.P.; Harder-Ruckstuhl, M. Management of Benign Inverted Sinonasal Papilloma Avoiding External Approaches. *J. Laryngol. Otol.* **2007**, *121*, 548–554. [CrossRef]
Kamel, R.H.; Abdel Fattah, A.F.; Awad, A.G. Origin Oriented Management of Inverted Papilloma of the Frontal Sinus. *Rhinology* **2012**, *50*, 262–268. [CrossRef] [PubMed]
Karligkiotis, A.; Pistochini, A.; Turri-Zanoni, M.; Terranova, P.; Volpi, L.; Battaglia, P.; Bignami, M.; Castelnuovo, P. Endoscopic Endonasal Orbital Transposition to Expand the Frontal Sinus Approaches. *Am. J. Rhinol. Allergy* **2015**, *29*, 449–456. [CrossRef]
Kim, Y.M.; Kim, H.S.; Park, J.Y.; Koo, B.S.; Park, Y.H.; Rha, K.S. External vs. Endoscopic Approach for Inverted Papilloma of the Sino-Nasal Cavities: A Retrospective Study of 136 Cases. *Acta Otolaryngol.* **2008**, *128*, 909–914. [CrossRef] [PubMed]
Lawson, W.; Ho, B.T.; Shaari, C.M.; Biller, H.F. Inverted Papilloma: A Report of 112 Cases. *Laryngoscope* **1995**, *105*, 282–288. [CrossRef] [PubMed]
Lawson, W.; Kaufman, M.R.; Biller, H.F. Treatment Outcomes in the Management of Inverted Papilloma: An Analysis of 160 Cases. *Laryngoscope* **2003**, *113*, 1548–1556. [CrossRef]
Lombardi, D.; Tomenzoli, D.; Buttà, L.; Bizzoni, A.; Farina, D.; Sberze, F.; Karligkiotis, A.; Castelnuovo, P.; Nicolai, P. Limitations and Complications of Endoscopic Surgery for Treatment for Sinonasal Inverted Papilloma: A Reassessment after 212 Cases. *Head Neck* **2011**, *33*, 1154–1161. [CrossRef]
Minni, A.; Gera, R.; Bulgheroni, C.; Ralli, M.; Cialente, F.; Candelori, F.; Mevio, N.; Dragonetti, A. Endoscopic Resection of Sinonasal Inverted Papilloma: A Multivariate Retrospective Analysis of Factors Affecting Recurrence and Persistence. *Ear Nose Throat J.* **2021**, *100*, 542s–548s. [CrossRef]
Minovi, A.; Kollert, M.; Draf, W.; Bockmühl, U. Inverted Papilloma: Feasibility of Endonasal Surgery and Long-Term Results of 87 Cases. *Rhinology* **2006**, *44*, 205–210.
Nygren, A.; Kiss, K.; von Buchwald, C.; Bilde, A. Rate of Recurrence and Malignant Transformation in 88 Cases with Inverted Papilloma between 1998-2008. *Acta Otolaryngol.* **2016**, *136*, 333–336. [CrossRef]

41. Pietrobon, G.; Karligkiotis, A.; Turri-Zanoni, M.; Fazio, E.; Battaglia, P.; Bignami, M.; Castelnuovo, P. Surgical Managemen Inverted Papilloma Involving the Frontal Sinus: A Practical Algorithm for Treatment Planning. *Acta Otorhinolaryngol. Ital.* **2** *39*, 28–39. [CrossRef]
42. Promsopa, C.; Thanahirunrojh, S. Surgical Outcomes of Sinonasal Inverted Papillomas in Songklanagarind Hospital. *J. M Assoc. Thai* **2015**, *98*, 1209–1214. [PubMed]
43. Sautter, N.B.; Citardi, M.J.; Batra, P.S. Minimally Invasive Resection of Frontal Recess/Sinus Inverted Papilloma. *Am. J. Otolary* **2007**, *28*, 221–224. [CrossRef] [PubMed]
44. Sciarretta, V.; Fernandez, I.J.; Farneti, P.; Pasquini, E. Endoscopic and Combined External-Transnasal Endoscopic Approach for Treatment of Inverted Papilloma: Analysis of 110 Cases. *Eur. Arch. Otorhinolaryngol.* **2014**, *271*, 1953–1959. [CrossRef] [PubM
45. Sham, C.L.; van Hasselt, C.A.; Chow, S.M.W.; Lee, D.L.Y.; Cho, R.H.W.; Woo, J.K.S.; Tong, M.C.F. Frontal Inverted Papillomas 25-Year Study. *Laryngoscope* **2020**, *130*, 1622–1628. [CrossRef]
46. Takahashi, Y.; Shoji, F.; Katori, Y.; Hidaka, H.; Noguchi, N.; Abe, Y.; Kakuta, R.K.; Suzuki, T.; Suzuki, Y.; Ohta, N.; et al. Endosc Surgical Management of Sinonasal Inverted Papilloma Extending to Frontal Sinuses. *Otolaryngol. Pol.* **2016**, *70*, 26–32. [CrossR
47. Verillaud, B.; Le Clerc, N.; Blancal, J.P.; Guichard, J.P.; Kania, R.; Classe, M.; Herman, P. Mucocele Formation after Surg Treatment of Inverted Papilloma of the Frontal Sinus Drainage Pathway. *Am. J. Rhinol. Allergy* **2016**, *30*, 181–184. [CrossRef]
48. Von Buchwald, C.; Larsen, A.S. Endoscopic Surgery of Inverted Papillomas under Image Guidance—A Prospective Study o Consecutive Cases at a Danish University Clinic. *Otolaryngol. Head Neck Surg.* **2005**, *132*, 602–607. [CrossRef]
49. Yoon, B.N.; Batra, P.S.; Citardi, M.J.; Roh, H.J. Frontal Sinus Inverted Papilloma: Surgical Strategy Based on the Site of Attachm *Am. J. Rhinol. Allergy* **2009**, *23*, 337–341. [CrossRef]
50. Yu, S.; Grose, E.; Lee, D.J.; Wu, V.; Pellarin, M.; Lee, J.M. Evaluation of Inverted Papilloma Recurrence Rates and Fact Associated Recurrence after Endoscopic Surgical Resection: A Retrospective Review. *J. Otolaryngol. Head Neck Surg.* **2023**, *52* [CrossRef]
51. Zhang, L.; Han, D.; Wang, C.; Ge, W.; Zhou, B. Endoscopic Management of the Inverted Papilloma with Attachment to the Fro Sinus Drainage Pathway. *Acta Otolaryngol.* **2008**, *128*, 561–568. [CrossRef] [PubMed]
52. Delaine, E.; Gorostidi, F.; Guilcher, P.; Lambercy, K.; Litzistorf, Y.; Bron, L.; Reinhard, A. Risk Factors for Recurrence after Surg Resection of Sinonasal Inverted Papilloma. *Int. Arch. Otorhinolaryngol.* **2024**, *28*, e568–e573. [CrossRef] [PubMed]
53. Woodworth, B.A.; Bhargave, G.A.; Palmer, J.N.; Chiu, A.G.; Cohen, N.A.; Lanza, D.C.; Bolger, W.E.; Kennedy, D.W. Clin Outcomes of Endoscopic and Endoscopic-Assisted Resection of Inverted Papillomas: A 15-Year Experience. *Am. J. Rhinol.* **2** *21*, 591–600. [CrossRef]
54. SamimiArdestani, S. The Characteristics of Sinonasal Inverted Papilloma and Recurrence Factors: An Analysis of 207 Ca *World J. Otorhinolaryngol. Head Neck Surg.* **2024**, 1–6. [CrossRef]
55. Busquets, J.M.; Hwang, P.H. Endoscopic Resection of Sinonasal Inverted Papilloma: A Meta-Analysis. *Otolaryngol.-Head N Surg.* **2006**, *134*, 476–482. [CrossRef] [PubMed]
56. Kim, J.S.; Kwon, S.H. Recurrence of Sinonasal Inverted Papilloma Following Surgical Approach: A Meta-Analysis. *Laryngosc* **2017**, *127*, 52–58. [CrossRef]
57. Bastier, P.L.; de Gabory, L. Design and Assessment of an Anatomical Diagram for Sinonasal Malignant Tumour Resect *Rhinology* **2016**, *54*, 361–367. [CrossRef]
58. Wang, Y.; An, Y.; Zhao, C.; Dong, R.; Cheng, F. Attachment-Oriented Endoscopic Treatment of Inverted Papilloma Involving Frontal Sinus/Recess. *J. Craniofac. Surg.* **2020**, *31*, e778–e781. [CrossRef]
59. Yan, Y.; Liu, Y.; Tao, J.; Li, Z.; Qu, X.; Guo, J.; Xian, J. Preoperative Prediction of Malignant Transformation of Sinonasal Inver Papilloma Using MR Radiomics. *Front. Oncol.* **2022**, *12*, 870544. [CrossRef]
60. Lawson, W.; Ho, Y. Open Frontal Sinus Surgery: A Lost Art. *Otolaryngol. Clin. N. Am.* **2016**, *49*, 1067–1089. [CrossRef]

Journal of
Personalized Medicine

MDPI

cle

ɔmprehensive Management of Cocaine-Induced Midline estructive Lesions: A Young-IfOS Consensus

erto Maria Saibene [1,2], Letizia Nitro [1,2], Florent Carsuzaa [1,3,4], Mihaela Alexandru [1,5,6], Vincent Bedarida [1,7], tteo Di Bari [1,8], Léa Fath [1,9,10], Ainhoa Garcia-Lliberos [1,11], Margaux Legré [1,12], David Lobo-Duro [1,13,14], onino Maniaci [1,15], Thomas Radulesco [1,16,17], Leigh Sowerby [1,18], Neil Tan [1,19], Manuel Tucciarone [1,20], ir Vandersteen [1,21,22], Valentin Favier [1,23,24] and Maxime Fieux [1,25,*]

1 Young Otolaryngologists-International Federation of Otorhinolaryngological Societies (Yo-IFOS), F-75000 Paris, France; alberto.saibene@gmail.com (A.M.S.); letizia.nitro@gmail.com (L.N.); florent.carsuzaa@gmail.com (F.C.); mihaela.dana.alexandru@gmail.com (M.A.); vincent.bedarida@gmail.com (V.B.); mattediba@gmail.com (M.D.B.); lea.fath@chru-strasbourg.fr (L.F.); ainhoa.glliberos@gmail.com (A.G.-L.); margauxlegre@gmail.com (M.L.); david.lobo@scsalud.es (D.L.-D.); tnmaniaci29@gmail.com (A.M.); thomas.radulesco@gmail.com (T.R.); leigh.sowerby@gmail.com (L.S.); neil.tan@nhs.net (N.T.); tucciaronemanuel@hotmail.it (M.T.); vandersteen.c@chu-nice.fr (C.V.)

2 Otolaryngology Unit, ASST Santi Paolo E Carlo, Department of Health Sciences, Università Degli Studi Di Milano, F-20133 Milan, Italy

3 Service ORL, Chirurgie Cervico-Maxillo-Faciale et Audiophonologie, Centre Hospitalier Universitaire de Poitiers, F-86000 Poitiers, France

4 Laboratoire Inflammation Tissus Epithéliaux et Cytokines (LITEC), Université de Poitiers, 86000 Poitiers, France

5 Service d'Orl et Chirurgie Cervico-Faciale, Assistance Publique-Hôpitaux de Paris (AP-HP), Université Paris-Saclay, Hôpital Bicêtre, F-94270 le Kremlin-Bicêtre, France

6 Sorbonne Université, Institut National de la Santé et de la Recherche Médicale, Hôpital Armand-Trousseau, F-75012 Paris, France

7 Otolaryngology-Head and Neck Surgery Department, Hôpital Lariboisière, Assistance Publique-Hôpitaux de Paris, F-75010 Paris, France

8 Otolaryngology Department, Hôpitaux Universitaires Pitié Salpêtrière-Charles Foix, Assistance Publique-Hôpitaux de Paris, F-75013 Paris, France

9 Service d'ORL, de Chirurgie Cervico Faciale, Hôpital de Hautepierre, Hôpitaux Universitaires de Strasbourg, F-67200 Strasbourg, France

10 Unité Inserm 1121, Biomatériaux et Bioingénierie, F-67000 Strasbourg, France

11 ENT Department, Valencia General University, F-46014 Valencia, Spain

12 Service ORL et Chirurgie Cervico-Faciale, Institut Arthur Vernes, F-75006 Paris, France

13 Otolaryngology Department, Hospital Universitario Marques de Valdecilla, F-39008 Santander, Spain

14 Valdecilla Biomedical Research Institute (IDIVAL), F-39008 Santander, Spain

15 Department of Otolaryngology, Kore University, F-94100 Enna, Italy

16 ENT-Head and Neck Surgery Department, APHM, La Conception University Hospital, Aix Marseille University, F-13005 Marseille, France

17 CNRS, IUSTI, Aix Marseille University, F-13007 Marseille, France

18 Department of Otolaryngology-Head and Neck Surgery, Western University, London, ON N6A 3K7, Canada

19 Department of Otolaryngology, Royal Cornwall Hospital, Truro TR1 3LJ, UK

20 Department of Otolaryngology and Head and Neck Surgery, University Hospital of Jerez, F-11407 Cádiz, Spain

21 Institut Universitaire de La Face et du Cou, Centre Hospitalier Universitaire de Nice, F-06000 Nice, France

22 Unité de Recherche Clinique de Nice Côte d'Azur (UR2CA), Université Côte d'Azur, F-06000 Nice, France

23 Département d'ORL, Chirurgie Cervico Faciale et Maxillo-Faciale, Hôpital Gui de Chauliac, CHU de Montpellier, F-34295 Montpellier, France

24 Research-Team ICAR, Laboratory of Computer Science, Robotics and Microelectronics of Montpellier (LIRMM), University Montpellier, French National Centre for Scientific Research (CNRS), F-34295 Montpellier, France

25 Hospices Civils de Lyon, Centre Hospitalier Lyon Sud, Service d'ORL, D'otoneurochirurgie et de Chirurgie Cervico-Faciale, F-69495 Pierre Bénite, France

* Correspondence: maxime.fieux@chu-lyon.fr; Tel.: +33-472666415

 https://doi.org/10.3390/jpm15060231

Abstract: Background: Recreational nasal cocaine use (RNCU) presents a significant challenge for rhinologists due to cocaine-induced midline destructive lesions (CIMDLs). This clinical consensus statement (CCS) offers guidelines for diagnosing, assessing, and managing both proven and suspected cases of CIMDL (including those without a prior RNCU history). It aims to support clinicians in addressing these complex cases effectively. **Methods:** An international, multidisciplinary panel of 18 specialists employed a three-round modified Delphi-method survey to evaluate statements covering CIMDL management issues such as definition, clinical evaluation and diagnosis, initial management approaches, and surgical management of complications and reconstructions. This study primarily targets otorhinolaryngologists. **Results:** Out of 44 evaluated statements, 20 achieved strong consensus, 20 reached consensus, 3 approached near-consensus, and 1 failed to achieve consensus. Consensus-covered areas included the definition of CIMDL, clinical evaluations, first-line management, and management of complications. However, reconstructive techniques remained a contentious topic. **Conclusions:** In the absence of extensive data, this CCS establishes a management framework for CIMDL, significantly bridging a knowledge gap. It highlights the need for standardized assessments, multidisciplinary cooperation, and customized follow-up care for patients with CIMDL. Considering the widespread use of cocaine, physicians should consistently consider the possibility of RNCU when encountering chronic inflammatory lesions in the sinonasal tract.

Keywords: endoscopy; computed tomography; recreational cocaine use; differential diagnosis; granulomatous disease; cocaine-induced midline destructive lesion

1. Introduction

Estimating the prevalence of cocaine snorting, or recreational nasal cocaine use (RNCU), is complex due to its illegal status and potential survey underreporting. The United Nations Office on Drugs and Crime's World Drug Report 2021 estimated that around 19 million people globally, or 0.4% of the population aged 15–64, used cocaine in any form during 2019 [1]. In Europe, the European Monitoring Centre for Drugs and Drug Addiction reported that 2.3% of individuals aged 15–34 years used cocaine in 2022 [2]. The lifetime prevalence of RNCU is around 3.9% in Brazil, with European rates varying from 0.3% to 11% [2,3]. This makes RNCU notably significant due to the array of potential health symptoms it can induce.

Chronic RNCU (defined as use for at least 6 months, administered at least 4 times a month) can lead to severe health issues, including hyperthermia, cardiovascular problems, and neurological disorders [4], significantly affecting patients' quality of life [5]. From a rhinological perspective, RNCU can cause vasoconstriction and damage to the nasal mucosa, progressively harming the nasal perichondrium and periosteum. This often results in a damaging condition known as cocaine-induced midline destructive lesions (CIMDLs) [6]. Adulterants in cocaine, such as levamisole, may exacerbate these destructive effects through autoimmune responses [6,7]. CIMDLs can vary from minor septal perforations to severe skull base damage, with the Nitro et al. classification system developed to categorize these injuries [5]. Early signs like septal perforations (Nitro et al. classification grade 1) often present diagnostic challenges as they are not specific to RNCU [8].

Given the scarcity of research specifically addressing the diagnosis, assessment, and management of CIMDL, predominantly retrospective, an expert-led clinical consensus statement (CCS) has been developed. This CCS utilizes a modified Delphi process to provide management guidelines based on the best available evidence for proven and suspected CIMDL, addressing common and complex clinical scenarios.

2. Materials and Methods

This CCS was developed according to the modified Delphi protocol by Rosenfeld et al. [9]. The French Ethic Committee of otorhinolaryngology has issued a favorable decision (n° 2024-03-035-VF) to conduct the study.

2.1. Panelists and Scope of Consensus Statement

The Delphi committee was made up of 18 voluntary members of the Young Otolaryngologist section of the International Federation of Otorhinolaryngological Societies (Yo-IFOS) rhinology research group from five countries across Europe and North America. The YO-IFOS research group is an invitation-only group, whose members are selected by the elected scientific committee of the YO-IFOS among worldwide board-certified otolaryngologists younger than 45 years old based on the extent and impact of their scientific production. The group is further subdivided according to members' subspecialties. As is the case for this CCS, members are free to propose new projects and participate in proposals according to their areas of expertise (though one completed proposal and two participations every 24 months are required to retain membership). The core development team included a chairperson (VF), a vice-chairperson (LN), and a methodologist (AMS). VF and LN were selected as leading and proposing the research project, and AMS due to their extensive experience both in CIMDLs and in Delphi consensuses. An additional team comprising two rhinologists randomly chosen among panelists (FC and MF) enhanced the initial draft of the CCS. These rhinologists joined on a voluntary basis from the Yo-IFOS or were recommended by the group as experts in CIMDLs. The authors reported no conflicts of interest. The CCS was designed to provide specific recommendations for managing CIMDLs.

2.2. Systematic Literature Review

An equation research systematic review adhering to PRISMA guidelines was carried out across the MEDLINE, EMBASE, Scopus, and Web of Science databases to explore management strategies for CIMDLs. Comprehensive search terms including both the acronym and full definition of CIMDLs, along with 'cocaine' and related terms pertaining to the paranasal sinuses and nose, were employed on 19 July 2023. This search aimed to identify studies published in English, Italian, German, French, or Spanish that presented data derived from human participants.

The basic search string was (cocaine and (midline OR nose OR turbinate OR concha OR nasal OR palate OR "skull base" OR sinus OR septum)) OR CIMDL OR "cocaine-induced midline destructive lesion".

Owing to the scarcity of high-quality research available, the scope of the systematic review was broadened beyond the initially advised parameters for CCSs, which typically encompass guidelines and systematic reviews [9]. It was expanded to incorporate randomized clinical trials relevant to the subject, adopting a methodological approach that aligns with other recent CCSs in the field of head and neck research [10,11].

Based on the search equation and inclusion criteria set up initially to perform a systematic review, 23 articles were included [5,6,12–32], representing the highest-quality evidence available on the subject. However, as most of the studies were only descriptive low-level-of-evidence (level 4 or 5) studies without any control group, a systematic review could not be performed, justifying the choice of a CCS methodology. This compilation was shared with all authors for review over a period of one month. Figure 1 illustrates the selection process of these articles using a PRISMA flow chart. The authors involved were invited to suggest any additional literature they deemed crucial to the CCS's breadth. Consequently, one more article was added to this collection [33].

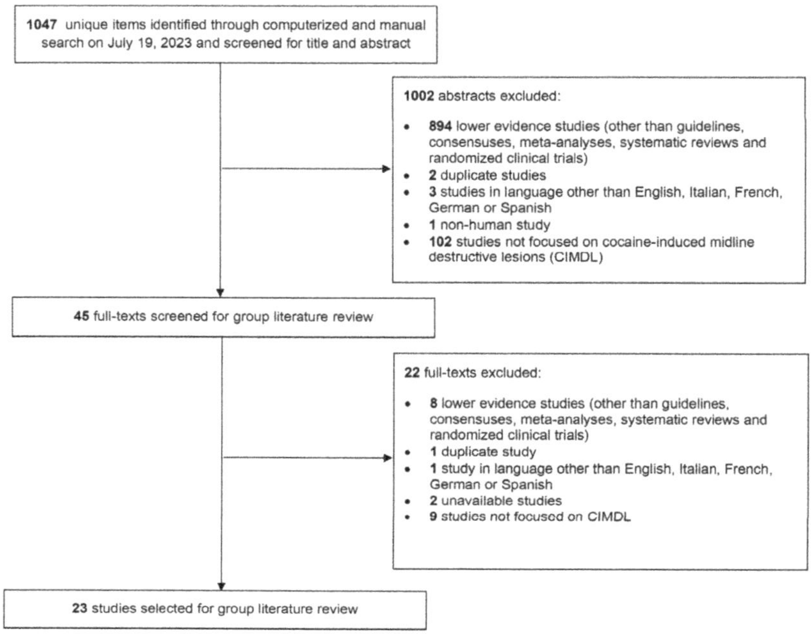

Figure 1. PRISMA-style flow chart of the article selection process for the systematic review of the literature about cocaine-induced midline destructive lesion (CIMDL) management.

2.3. Clinical Statement Development and Modified Delphi Survey

Guided by the literature review and the objectives of the CCS, the chair and assistant chair crafted the initial clinical statements for the survey. These statements were then elaborated, refined, and extended through discussions with the methodologist. Following this, the secondary development group evaluated the preliminary draft prior to initiating the Delphi rounds.

The statements were shaped by insights from the literature review and the development group's understanding of key clinical scenarios, resulting in a comprehensive 44-statement survey. This survey was disseminated to the authors via Google Forms (Google LLC, Mountain View, CA, USA). Participants were asked to fill out the survey anonymously, using a one-time link and a personal identification number (PIN) to prevent duplicate responses and maintain anonymity. The coordination of PINs was managed by a single coordinator, who was not directly involved in the CCS, ensuring the anonymity of panelist responses. The authors rated each statement on a 9-point Likert scale ranging from strongly disagree (1) to strongly agree (9). According to Rosenfeld [9], the outcomes for each statement were categorized as follows: strong consensus was achieved if the mean score was ≥8.00 without any outliers (an outlier being a rating that deviated by 2 or more points from the mean in either direction); consensus was noted if the mean score was ≥7.00 with no more than one outlier; near-consensus was indicated by a mean score of ≥6.50 with no more than two outliers; all other responses were categorized as having no consensus.

All panelists were asked to provide comments explaining their refusal or proposing new statements to be implemented in the following rounds.

3. Results

All panelists participated in three Delphi rounds. After the initial round, consensus levels were as follows: 4 out of 44 statements achieved strong consensus, 9 reached consensus, 16 reached near-consensus, and 15 did not reach consensus. The 31 statements that did not achieve at least consensus were revised for greater inclusivity and clarity, based on anonymous feedback from the authors. The revised second round included these 31 statements, resulting in 5 achieving strong consensus, 6 reaching consensus, 10 achieving near-consensus, and 10 still lacking consensus. Following further revisions, a third and final round was conducted with 20 statements, of which 11 statements achieved strong consensus, 5 reached consensus, 3 reached near-consensus, and 1 did not achieve consensus. Overall, from the total of 44 statements, 20 reached strong consensus, 20 reached consensus, 3 reached near-consensus, and 1 failed to reach consensus after all rounds. The progression of the statements from the first round to their finalized versions is detailed in Appendix A. The results of the Delphi process for all statements, including their mean scores, median scores, score ranges, and the number of outliers, are documented in Tables 1–5. Definitions of CIMDLs are shown in Table 1, clinical evaluation and diagnosis in Table 2, first-line management in Table 3, and surgical management of complications in Table 4, while statements with no consensus are in Table 5.

Table 1. Statements and results from the Delphi process for items reaching consensus or strong consensus: disease definition.

em .o.	Statement	Mean	Median	Min	Max	Outliers	Result	Delphi Round
.1	CIMDLs are defined as any structural lesion of the sinonasal complex ascertained in the context of a toxicological screening- or patient history-confirmed cocaine-snorting habit	7.44	7.5	1	9	1	consensus	1
.2	CIMDLs can refer both to sinonasal and palatal lesions due to cocaine snorting	8.83	9	8	9	0	strong consensus	1
.3	CIMDL diagnosis should not rely on auto-antibody testing, which might result positive or negative results in CIMDL patients	8.50	9	7	9	0	strong consensus	3

Table 2. Statements and results from the Delphi process for items reaching consensus or strong consensus: clinical evaluation and diagnosis.

em lo.	Statement	Mean	Median	Min	Max	Outliers	Result	Delphi Round
.1	Clinical assessment of potential CIMDLs should include face examination, anterior rhinoscopy, oral examination, and nasal endoscopy	8.61	9	7	9	0	strong consensus	1
.2	The degree of nasal structures involvement can be assessed via the Nitro et al. classification of CIMDLs	8.44	9	5	9	0	consensus	1

Table 2. *Cont.*

Item No.	Statement	Mean	Median	Min	Max	Outliers	Result	Delp Rour
2.3	Differential diagnoses for CIMDLs include vasculitis (including but not limited to granulomatosis with polyangiitis), T-cell or NK/T lymphoma, infectious disease (including, but not limited to, syphilis, leishmaniasis, yaws, leprosy, tuberculosis, and actinomycosis), chronic intestinal bowel disease (e.g., Crohn's disease), chronic use of vasoconstrictor drugs, rhinotillexomania, trauma, other recreational intranasal drug use (amphetamine, acetaminophen–oxycodone), IgG4-related disease, relapsing polychondritis, rhinoscleroma, sclerosing orbital pseudotumor, and iatrogeny	8.50	9	6	9	1	consensus	2
2.4	In the case of isolated septal perforations, cocaine-snorting habits should be investigated in the patient history as well as traumas, prior nasal or nose-involving procedures (including radiotherapy and intranasal oxygen therapy), prolonged intranasal vasoconstrictor use, picking habits or history of foreign bodies, known infectious diseases, and known autoimmune disease or vasculitis	8.67	9	7	9	0	strong consensus	2
2.5	If an isolated septal perforation is not identified as a CIMDL, but no other causative factor can be identified, a biopsy should be considered with the patient, and—if ruled out—a personalized follow-up should be planned to check for lesion evolution, possibly with measurement and clinical image documentation	8.33	9	7	9	0	strong consensus	2
2.6	Patients presenting with a potential CIMDL grade II or higher, without a history of cocaine-snorting, should undergo a complete workup including serology (ESR, ANA, C-ANCA—with immunofluorescence for NPO and PR3 if positive—IgG4, and rheumatoid factor), rheumatology/internal medicine and infectious disease consultation, and nasal biopsy	7.78	9	3	9	1	consensus	1

Table 2. *Cont.*

em No.	Statement	Mean	Median	Min	Max	Outliers	Result	Delphi Round
.9	In patients presenting with a potential CIMDL without a history of cocaine snorting and with negative workup and cocaine testing results, other less common snorting substances can be assessed (e.g., methamphetamine, heroin)	7.89	8	5	9	1	consensus	1
.1	Destructive midline lesions due to nasal administration of non-cocaine recreational drugs (e.g., amphetamine, acetaminophen–oxycodone) can be clinically managed as CIMDLs	7.83	9	1	9	1	consensus	3
.11	Patients presenting with a potential CIMDL and confirming a cocaine-snorting habit should be considered de facto CIMDL patients and receive adequate care and follow-up, though biopsies might still be discussed with the patient to rule out differentials	8.06	9	3	9	1	consensus	3
.12	Enlarging isolated septal perforations in non-CIMDL patients should undergo a complete workup including serology (ESR, ANA, C-ANCA—with immunofluorescence for NPO and PR3 if positive—IgG4, and rheumatoid factor) and nasal biopsy (for histological and microbiological analysis), considering rheumatology, internal medicine, or infectious disease referral according to results	8.67	9	7	9	0	strong consensus	3
.13	Patients reporting complete cessation of RNCU with an increase in CIMDL involvement at follow-up should undergo a complete workup including serology (ESR, ANA, C-ANCA, and rheumatoid factor), rheumatology/internal medicine/infectious disease consultation, and nasal biopsy (both for histological and microbiological analysis)	8.56	9	7	9	0	strong consensus	3

Table 2. *Cont.*

Item No.	Statement	Mean	Median	Min	Max	Outliers	Result	Delphi Round
2.14	In case of an increase in CIMDL involvement at follow-up in patients reporting stopping recreational cocaine use, a drug test can be considered	8.22	9	5	9	1	consensus	1
2.15	Patients with potential CIMDLs, especially with negative workup, can be offered a nasal mucosal biopsy under local or general anesthesia to assist with diagnosis	7.94	9	3	9	1	consensus	3

Table 3. Statements and results from the Delphi process for items reaching consensus or strong consensus: first-line management of CIMDL patients.

Item No.	Statement	Mean	Median	Min	Max	Outliers	Result	Delphi Round
3.1	CIMDL patients could be encouraged to meet a specialist in addiction medicine	8.39	9	3	9	1	consensus	2
3.2	Pain management in CIMDL patients should avoid strong opioids and rely on an addiction medicine service and/or pain medicine services in case of uncontrolled pain potentially requiring strong opioids	8.67	9	7	9	0	strong consensus	3
3.3	CIMDL patients must be advised that the only known method for halting lesion development is ceasing recreational nasal cocaine administration	8.61	9	7	9	0	strong consensus	1
3.4	Patients with CIMDL should be correctly informed that no "safe threshold" of cocaine usage prevents further CIMDL evolution	8.89	9	8	9	0	strong consensus	1
3.5	After proper information, any CIMDL patient can be offered a complete workup including serology (ESR, ANA, C-ANCA—with immunofluorescence for NPO and PR3 if positive—IgG4, and rheumatoid factor), rheumatology, internal medicine and/or infectious disease consultation, and nasal biopsy for increasing compliance to medical advice and therapies	8.22	8.5	7	9	0	strong consensus	3

Table 3. *Cont.*

m o.	Statement	Mean	Median	Min	Max	Outliers	Result	Delphi Round
.6	Grade II or higher CIMDL patients should always be assessed for signs of rhinosinusitis even in asymptomatic cases	8.50	9	6	9	1	consensus	2
.7	Grade III or higher CIMDL patients should be counseled for signs and symptoms of orbital or skull base complications and instructed to report to emergency department or specialty services promptly for evaluation	8.17	9	3	9	1	consensus	1
.8	Potential CIMDL extension and signs of secondary rhinosinusitis should be assessed with a CT scan, with the use of contrast medium limited to cases with suspected osteitis or osteonecrosis	8.00	9	3	9	1	consensus	1
.9	A baseline plain CT of the sinus (including the orbits and skull base) is recommended in patients presenting with CIMDL stage II or higher	8.56	9	7	9	0	strong consensus	2
.1	The use of MRI in CIMDLs should be limited to the evaluation of orbital, skull base, intracranial, or other soft tissue involvement	8.44	9	7	9	0	strong consensus	2
11	The impact of CIMDLs on sinonasal health should preferably be investigated with general nasal health questionnaires, though sinusitis-specific questionnaires may have a clinical and investigational role	8.39	9	5	9	1	consensus	3
12	CIMDL patients should be instructed to employ daily saline nasal lavages for nasal toilette and can employ nasal emollients for reducing crusting	8.44	9	3	9	1	consensus	1
13	Antibiotic therapy (systemic and/or topical) should be reserved for bacterial superinfections or osteitis, obtaining bone cultures in the latter scenario whenever possible	8.72	9	7	9	0	strong consensus	3
14	Endoscopic debridement of crusting and necrotic tissues during outpatient follow-up and/or high-volume nasal lavages can be offered to improve symptoms such as nasal obstruction and cacosmia	8.72	9	7	9	0	strong consensus	3

Table 3. *Cont.*

Item No.	Statement	Mean	Median	Min	Max	Outliers	Result	Delphi Round
3.15	CIMDL patients with palatal perforation can be offered palatal obturator prostheses as first-line management	8.11	9	3	9	1	consensus	1
3.16	Grade IV CIMDL patients should be proposed pneumococcal, haemophilus and meningococcal vaccine administration	8.22	9	3	9	1	consensus	3
3.17	Initial follow-up should be personalized and planned according to the CIMDL stage, considering more frequent visits to encourage RNCU cessation; in stable patients, a 6–12 month follow-up can be proposed up to 2–5 years after stopping cocaine snorting	8.28	9	7	9	0	strong consensus	3

Table 4. Statements and results from the Delphi process for items reaching consensus or strong consensus: surgical management of complications and reconstructions.

Item No.	Statement	Mean	Median	Min	Max	Outliers	Result	Delphi Round
4.1	CIMDL patients with symptoms and signs of rhinosinusitis should be proposed adequate medical and/or surgical treatment as per EPOS/ICAR:RS guidelines	8.44	9	5	9	2	consensus	2
4.2	Patients with signs and symptoms of osteitis or osteonecrosis should be offered debridement of necrotic tissue and adequate systemic antibiotic treatment guided by culture biopsy of a bony specimen and planned together with an infectious disease consultation	8.39	9	4	9	1	consensus	2
4.3	In patients with intraorbital complications from CIMDL, culture-guided antibiotic therapy should represent the first-line management, while endoscopic transnasal surgical debridement and drainage should be reserved for cases with sudden visual acuity reduction or loss of color perception, large or superior/lateral orbital abscesses, or failing medical therapy	8.44	9	7	9	0	strong consensus	3

Table 4. *Cont.*

Item No.	Statement	Mean	Median	Min	Max	Outliers	Result	Delphi Round
.4	Grade IV CIMDL without CSF leaks or intracranial complications should be managed conservatively (nasal toilette, antibiotics for superinfections, vaccine recommendarions)	8.72	9	7	9	0	strong consensus	3
.5	In fit-for-surgery grade IV CIMDL patients with ascertained CSF leaks, thorough debridement of necrotic tissues and prompt skull base reconstruction are recommended, and a neurosurgical consultation should be considered	8.67	9	7	9	0	strong consensus	3
.6	Patients with intracranial complications should be managed with culture-guided antibiotic therapy and/or surgical toilette via an endonasal or combined endonasal/craniotomy route, in a multidisciplinary rhinological and neurosurgical team, according to the specific complication	8.72	9	7	9	0	strong consensus	2
.7	Septal, nasal, and palatal reconstructions should not be performed in CIMDL patients unless the patient provides adequate motivation and proves cocaine use stopping by providing toxicological analyses covering at least 12 months	8.61	9	5	9	1	consensus	2

Table 5. Statements and results from the Delphi process for items not reaching consensus or strong consensus.

Item No.	Statement	Mean	Median	Min	Max	Outliers	Result	Delphi Round
.4	CIMDLs are due to RNCU only, while they are not related to medical nasal cocaine administration	7.61	9	1	9	2	near-consensus	3
2.7	Patients with suspected CIMDLs denying RNCU and with negative workup results should undergo a cocaine drug test for cocaine to adjust follow-up and treatment	7.83	9	3	9	3	no consensus	3
2.8	RNCU can be identified via urinary metabolites (3 to 15 days after use, also according to the administered dose) or hair analysis (up to 3 months after use)	8.28	9	3	9	2	near-consensus	3

Table 5. *Cont.*

Item No.	Statement	Mean	Median	Min	Max	Outliers	Result	Delphi Round
4.8	Reconstructions for CIMDL patients should be tailored to the patients; though pedicled flaps and vascularized free flaps usually represent the first option, autografts can still be considered, and allografts are usually adequate for a minority of patients	7.94	9	4	9	2	near-consensus	3

The top-scoring items for strong consensus were "Patients with CIMDL should be correctly informed that no "safe threshold" of cocaine usage prevents further CIMDL evolution" (mean score 8.89, median 9, no outliers) and "CIMDL can refer both to sinonasal and palatal lesions due to cocaine-snorting" (mean score 8.83, median 9, no outliers). A total of 29 out of 44 items recorded a median score of 9.

The lowest-scoring items, with mean scores of 7.61 and 7.44 and a median score of 7.5 for both, stated "CIMDL are due to RNCU only, while they are not related to nasal cocaine medical administration" and "CIMDL are defined as any structural lesion of the sinonasal complex ascertained in the context of a toxicological screening- or patient history-confirmed cocaine-snorting habit". The first of these two items was eventually removed from the CCS, while the second reached consensus.

4. Discussion

The multidisciplinary group of experts involved in the creation of this Delphi-method consensus statement has delineated a specific all-around management guideline for CIMDLs, thereby filling an important gap in the literature. Nitro et al. [5] proposed a classification system for CIMDLs according to the severity of the disease, which has been accepted by the panel. However, this initial article did not provide guidance on CIMDL management. Despite the scarcity of solid evidence, this CCS aims to improve outcomes and define a basic standard of care for CIMDL patients, focusing on complex diagnoses and recurrences. Therefore, this CCS can guide general otolaryngologists in managing challenging cases and allied specialties in referring patients for rhinology evaluation. A common need for standardization of CIDML care is evident from the frequent outliers in our peer-reviewed consensus statements, even in the disease definition sections. An overall management framework graphic representation based on the Nitro et al. classification of CIMDLs is reported in Figure 2.

4.1. Disease Definition

According to the panel, CIMDL is a clinical diagnosis based on the presence of at least one sinonasal lesion and a patient-confirmed history of RNCU. This resolution represents a significant step towards simplifying the diagnosis. It follows more modern views on the subject [6,31], in contrast to older positions that required at least two lesions for CIMDL diagnosis [34]. According to our CCS, there is no need to perform systematic auto-antibody testing when the clinical history is clear, given the inconclusive significance of a positive test in RNCU patients [6,35–37]. RNCU-induced mucosal membrane alteration leads to CIMDLs, possibly affecting the palate, the sinonasal complex, and its neighboring structures such as the orbits or the skull base [30,38]. This potential involvement justifies performing a complete facial, nasal, and oral examination and the use of anterior rhinoscopy and nasal endoscopy. Interestingly, the CCS failed to reach a consensus threshold regarding the use of medical nasal cocaine administration as a cause of CIMDLs. Medically administered cocaine has a known risk of inducing nasal lesions [18], but at present, CIMDLs should remain confined to RNCU patients, given the peculiar disease course. It is worth remembering that the recommended therapeutic topical dose of cocaine for local anesthesia is 1.5 mg/kg [39], and there is a 35% systemic absorption of topical nasal cocaine use [40], with some reports of cardiac complications following medical nasal administration [41]. By contrast, such a dose is far from RNCU exposure, with daily "runs" of 1000 mg and over [26], while recent studies have proven efficacy and safety profiles when medical cocaine is properly administered [42]. It is worth noting that medical cocaine use is declining in most regions [43], further reducing the potential for iatrogenic cocaine-induced lesions. A challenge remains for the definition of CIMDLs when patients have withdrawn from any RCNU in the past few months. When facing an isolated septal perforation, both the duration of the abstinence from drug use and the clinical characteristics of the midline lesion should be considered by physicians as time only is not reliable enough. As suggested in statements 2.3, 2.4 and 2.5, if there was RCNU within the previous years but without any recent consumption, the observation of an isolated septal perforation with good healing (neither crusting nor inflammation) could suggest a CIMDL. However, if there was active inflammation or crusting regarding the perforation, then further explorations should be run and a differential diagnosis should be considered.

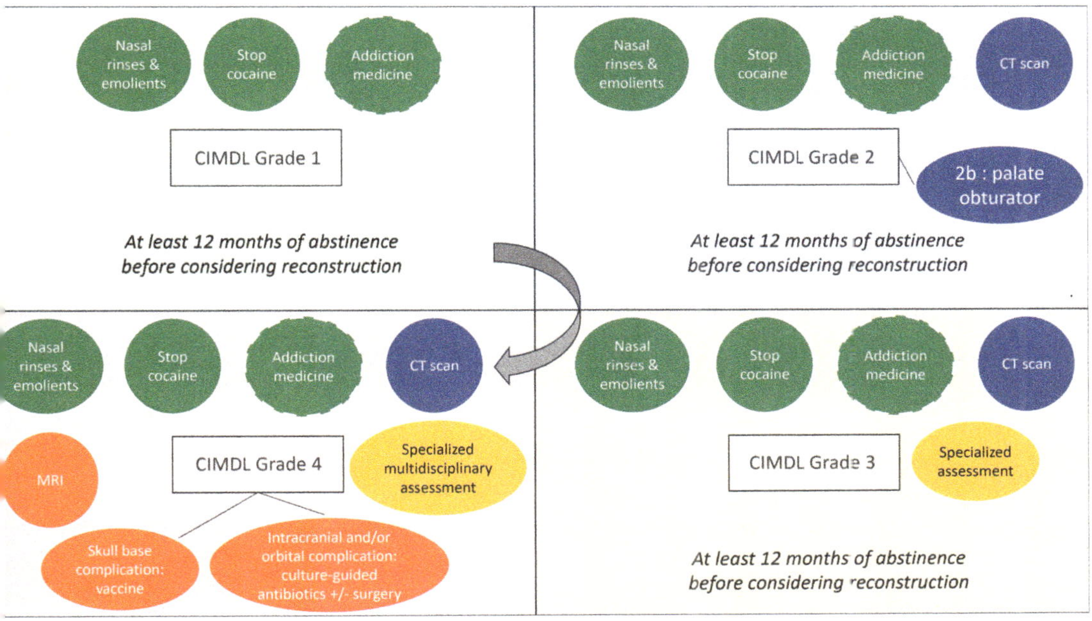

Figure 2. PRIMSA flow chart of the literature. Overview of the cocaine-induced midline destructive lesion (CIMDL) management proposed according to Nitro et al.'s classification grades. Dotted circles represent options to discuss with patients on a case-by-case basis (CT, computed tomography; MRI, magnetic resonance imaging).

4.2. Clinical Evaluation and Diagnosis

Given its scientific background and the lack of other significant options, our CCS suggests using the Nitro et al. classification for grading CIMDLs. This classification was developed according to a literature review to standardize the report of sinonasal and palatal anatomical structure involvement [5]. It describes four stages of increasing CIMDL anatomical structure involvement: nasal septum (grade 1), inferior part of the lateral nasal wall and hard palate (grade 2a and 2b), ethmoid and sphenoid region (grade 3), and orbit or skull base involvement (grade 4).

Differential diagnosis is one of the most difficult aspects of CIMDL management explored in this CCS. In a considerable number of cases, midline destructive lesions are not linked to a declared history of cocaine snorting and/or caused by RNCU [44]. According to the CCS, a patient with grade 2 or higher CIMDL with no history of drug snorting should undergo a complete workup to search for autoimmune, infection, or tumoral lesions using serology (ESR, ANA, C-ANCA—with immunofluorescence for NPO and PR3 if positive—IgG4, and rheumatoid factor), rheumatology/internal medicine and infectious disease consultation, and nasal biopsy. Also, differential diagnosis should always include RNCU even if the patient initially denies it. In these cases, drug tests may be performed on-site using urine tests or hair tests based on the suspected delay between the last consumption and the visit. This diagnostic strategy could also be applied in case of enlarging septal perforation during the follow-up because idiopathic midline lesions are rare [27]. To improve sensibility, panelists proposed to perform a biopsy, either under local or general anesthesia according to surgeons' and patients' preferences. It is important to remember that any crusted lesion of the nasal mucosa may be cancer, but some lesions such as primary sinonasal lymphoma can be challenging to diagnose even at the biopsy level and often require collecting multiple samples [45].

For patients presenting with non-otherwise-explained rhinitis [46] or an isolated septal perforation (grade 1 equivalent in the Nitro et al. classification), RNCU should be investigated as well as the use of intranasal vasoconstrictors, picking habits, and traumatic, infectious or autoimmune history. Of course, when there is any suspicion of tumoral involvement in the mucosa, a biopsy should be performed. The choice of cocaine tests (urinary metabolite analysis and/or hair analysis) in patients with potential CIMDLs has been debated and only achieved a near-consensus in the third CCS round [47], with panelists questioning the timing, modalities, and appropriateness of tests. Cocaine testing was proposed to confirm CIMDLs in patients who denied RNCU [48]. While this approach could be used on a case-by-case basis to offer patients a targeted support approach to recover from addiction, it is important to remember that rare false positives exist and might lead to wrong medical decisions [49]. Interestingly, levamisole can also be detected in urine tests, and it could be relevant to include it in the drugs usually screened to assess the risk of induced vasculitis [50]. In the case of non-cocaine-induced midline lesions, other recreational nasal substance use should be assessed (e.g., heroin [51] or methamphetamine [52]) and—if present—managed in a CIMDL-like framework.

At the other end of the severity spectrum, our CCS suggests that grade 3–4 CIMDL patients should be assessed for unknown orbital and skull base complications at presentation, as these patients require a specialized consultation with multidisciplinary clinical evaluation [53].

The use of a plain computed tomography (CT) of the sinuses was recommended in our CCS for CIMDL grade 2 patients or higher. In these cases, the CT scan can help to distinguish between grades 2–3 and 3–4 and point clinicians toward the correct specific management and follow-up plan. A CT scan with contrast should be reserved for suspected cases of osteitis/osteonecrosis, as the non-necrotic mucosa in people who use cocaine is extremely inflammatory and carries a risk of misinterpretation. Magnetic resonance imaging (MRI) must be proposed in case of orbit or skull base involvement to analyze the extension and infectious complications.

4.3. First-Line Management of CIMDL Patients

As CIMDLs are considered a complication of repeated RNCU, if allowed by local policies and medical facility availability, all patients should be encouraged to meet a specialist in addiction medicine for psychological [54] and pharmacological help [55]. In patients with painful symptoms due to CIMDLs, strong opioids should be avoided and intractable pain should be managed by an addiction/pain medicine service [56]. Furthermore, the CCS highlighted that there is no safe RNCU threshold and only complete RNCU cessation can block the disease progression [31]. Last, as is usually the case with complex conditions that transcend the boundaries of otolaryngological disease, our CCS suggests that follow-up should be personalized to encourage cocaine-snorting cessation.

4.4. Surgical Management of Complications and Reconstructions

In extreme cases, CIMDL extension can lead to orbital [57,58], skull base [38,59], or craniovertebral junction complications [60]. These potentially life-threatening infections require multidisciplinary management. When possible, the CCS favored a conservative treatment plan with nasal toilette, antibiotics for superinfection, and applying vaccine recommendations to prevent pneumococcal, Haemophilus, and meningococcal meningitis. The intracranial complications, such as infection or cerebrospinal fluid leaks, require collaboration with a neurosurgical team for a tailored surgical strategy. Skull base reconstruction after necrotic tissue debridement should be performed in ascertained cerebrospinal fluid leaks, using vascularized flaps when possible [61].

Apart from these life-threatening situations, reconstruction of a CIMDL defect—septum or palate—should only be proposed in patients with evidence of cessation of RNCU. Most groups performing reconstruction in CIMDL patients rely on repeated negative urine metabolite tests before considering surgery [62–64]. Our CCS recommended at least 12 months of abstinence, supported by toxicological analysis, and strong patient motivation to consider surgical repair. This threshold was suggested according to the literature where the sustained remission phase begins after 12 months of abstinence from drug use (Diagnostic and Statistical Manual of Mental Disorders fifth version criteria [65]). Indeed, evidence showed that the longer the duration of abstinence, the lower the risk of relapse. Unfortunately—but this is marginal concerning the scope of this CCS and suffers from the anecdotal nature of the pertaining literature—we failed to reach a consensus on the basic techniques that should be considered when treating CIMDL patients for reconstructive purposes.

The use of hyperbaric oxygen therapy to accelerate the pre- and postoperative reconstruction process may be an option to discuss but requires further evidence [66].

4.5. Limitations of the CCS

There were some limitations to the study due to its subjective nature. Authors tried to assess all relevant questions pertaining to CIMDLs, while focusing on sinonasal cavity lesions because they are responsible for almost all rhinology functional symptoms. Cocaine snorting may also affect the dorsal septum, nasal pyramid or lips with aesthetic complaints that were not assessed in the present study only involving rhinologists. A multidisciplinary CCS including input from rhinologists, maxillofacial surgeons, and plastic/reconstructive surgeons may be required to respond to the challenging management of nose deformities following cocaine snorting. However, while this CCS aims to provide guidance on common cases, it does not intend to replace the medical decision-making process, or to challenge the 12-step approach to control relapse in outpatient treatment for cocaine abuse, especially when physicians are facing heavily addicted users [67–69]. ENT specialists are neither experts nor referents in this field, which falls within the remit of addictology, and patients should be referred as recommended in paragraph 3.1: "CIMDL patients could be encouraged to meet a specialist in addiction medicine". At this stage, even though this CCS is a robust first step to guide physicians, many questions remain unanswered because of the difficult relationship of trust between physicians and drug users. Indeed, most drug addicts do not declare their consumption, and relapses are frequent. Unrepentant drug addicts, but also those who have difficulty weaning themselves off, should all use nasal rinses like any non-drug user suffering from rhinology symptoms [70]. It is also important to note that even if this study only focuses on cocaine abuse, assessing for multiple drug abuse is necessary as the latter can increase the complexity of CIMDL management. In these cases, a multidisciplinary approach with a thorough addictology assessment and close follow-up should be proposed, adapting the proposed statements on a case-by-case basis.

5. Conclusions

CIMDLs present significant obstacles in terms of diagnosis, addiction management, and therapeutic approach. This clinical consensus statement (CCS) recommends standardizing initial assessments and implementing customized follow-up plans, which should include multidisciplinary collaboration for more complex cases. Considering the prevalent use of cocaine in the general population, physicians should routinely consider cocaine snorting as a possible cause when encountering chronic inflammatory lesions in the sinonasal tract.

Author Contributions: A.M.S., V.F. and M.F.: consensus design, systematic review, statement draft and refinement, data collection, paper finalization; L.N., F.C. and M.F.: statement draft and refinements; all authors: consensus voting and analysis in all rounds, draft revision. All authors have read and agreed to the published version of the manuscript.

Funding: This research received no external funding.

Institutional Review Board Statement: This consensus statement does not involve human or animal data. The French Ethic Committee of otorhinolaryngology has is issued a favorable decision (n° 2024-03-035-VF) to conduct the study.

Informed Consent Statement: All panelists gave their written consent to participate in the study. Written informed consent has been obtained from the patient(s) to publish this paper.

Data Availability Statement: The data presented in this study are available on request from the corresponding author.

Acknowledgments: The authors would like to thank Eleonora Simini, medical student at Università degli Studi di Milano, Italy, for her invaluable help in coordinating emails and survey replies.

Conflicts of Interest: The authors declare no conflicts of interest.

Abbreviations

The following abbreviations are used in this manuscript:

RCNU	Recreational Cocaine Nasal Use
CIMDL	Cocaine-Induced Midline Destructive Lesions

Appendix A

Statements of the evolution across the three Delphi consensus rounds. (Blue: strong consensus; green: consensus; yellow: near-consensus; red: no consensus).

ferences

United Nations: Office on Drugs and Crime. World Drug Report 2021. Available online: https://www.unodc.org/unodc/en/data-and-analysis/wdr2021.html (accessed on 5 January 2024).
European Monitoring Centre for Drugs and Drug Addiction. European Drug Report 2023: Trends and Developments. Available online: https://www.emcdda.europa.eu/publications/european-drug-report/2023_en (accessed on 15 January 2024).
Abdalla, R.R.; Madruga, C.S.; Ribeiro, M.; Pinsky, I.; Caetano, R.; Laranjeira, R. Prevalence of cocaine use in Brazil: Data from the II Brazilian national alcohol and drugs survey (BNADS). *Addict. Behav.* **2014**, *39*, 297–301. [CrossRef]
Bravo, R.R.; Faria, A.C.; Brito-Da-Costa, A.M.; Carmo, H.; Mladěnka, P.; da Silva, D.D.; Remião, F.; Researchers, O.B.O.T.O. Cocaine: An Updated Overview on Chemistry, Detection, Biokinetics, and Pharmacotoxicological Aspects including Abuse Pattern. *Toxins* **2022**, *14*, 278. [CrossRef]
Nitro, L.; Pipolo, C.; Fadda, G.L.; Allevi, F.; Borgione, M.; Cavallo, G.; Felisati, G.; Saibene, A.M. Distribution of cocaine-induced midline destructive lesions: Systematic review and classification. *Eur. Arch. Otorhinolaryngol.* **2022**, *279*, 3257–3267. [CrossRef] [PubMed]
Trimarchi, M.; Bussi, M.; Sinico, R.A.; Meroni, P.; Specks, U. Cocaine-induced midline destructive lesions—An autoimmune disease? *Autoimmun. Rev.* **2013**, *12*, 496–500. [CrossRef]
Zwang, N.A.; Van Wagner, L.B.; Rose, S. A case of levamisole-induced systemic vasculitis and cocaine-induced midline destructive lesion: A case report. *J. Clin. Rheumatol.* **2011**, *17*, 197–200. [CrossRef] [PubMed]
Pereira, C.; Santamaría, A.; Langdon, C.; López-Chacón, M.; Hernández-Rodríguez, J.; Alobid, I. Nasoseptal Perforation: From Etiology to Treatment. *Curr. Allergy Asthma Rep.* **2018**, *18*, 5. [CrossRef] [PubMed]
Rosenfeld, R.M.; Nnacheta, L.C.; Corrigan, M.D. Clinical Consensus Statement Development Manual. *Otolaryngol. Head Neck Surg.* **2015**, *153* (Suppl. 2), S1–S14. [CrossRef] [PubMed]
Maniaci, A.; Calvo-Henriquez, C.; Cammaroto, G.; Garcia-Magan, C.; Garcia-Paz, V.; Iannella, G.; Jiménez-Huerta, I.; La Mantia, I.; Lechien, J.R.; Leong, S.C.; et al. Pediatric Inferior Turbinate Hypertrophy: Diagnosis and Management. A YO-IFOS Consensus Statement. *Laryngoscope* **2023**, *online ahead of print*. [CrossRef]
Saibene, A.M.; Allevi, F.; Calvo-Henriquez, C.; Dauby, N.; Dondossola, D.; Hervochon, R.; Lechien, J.R.; Lobo-Duro, D.; Locatello, L.G.; Maniaci, A.; et al. Comprehensive management of paranasal sinus fungus balls: A Young-IFOS consensus statement. *Int. Forum Allergy Rhinol.* **2023**, *13*, 877–885. [CrossRef]
Allbery, S.M.; Chaljub, G.; Cho, N.L.; Rassekh, C.H.; John, S.D.; Guinto, F.C. MR imaging of nasal masses. *Radiographics* **1995**, *15*, 1311–1327. [CrossRef]
Berman, M.; Paran, D.; Elkayam, O. Cocaine-Induced Vasculitis. *Rambam Maimonides Med. J.* **2016**, *31*, e0036. [CrossRef]
Dinis-Oliveira, R.J.; Carvalho, F.; Duarte, J.A.; Proença, J.B.; Santos, A.; Magalhães, T. Clinical and forensic signs related to cocaine abuse. *Curr. Drug Abus. Rev.* **2012**, *5*, 64–83.
Fuchs, H.A.; Tanner, S.B. Granulomatous disorders of the nose and paranasal sinuses. *Curr. Opin. Otolaryngol. Head Neck Surg.* **2009**, *17*, 23–27. [CrossRef]
Glauser, J.; Queen, J.R. An overview of non-cardiac cocaine toxicity. *J. Emerg. Med.* **2007**, *32*, 181–186. [CrossRef] [PubMed]
Gonik, N.J.; Bluth, M.H. Otolaryngology Concerns for Illicit and Prescription Drug Use. *Clin. Lab. Med.* **2016**, *36*, 745–752. [CrossRef] [PubMed]
Harper, S.J.; Jones, N.S. Cocaine: What role does it have in current ENT practice? A review of the current literature. *J. Laryngol. Otol.* **2006**, *120*, 808–811. [CrossRef] [PubMed]
Laudien, M. Orphan diseases of the nose and paranasal sinuses: Pathogenesis—clinic—therapy. *GMS Curr. Top. Otorhinolaryngol. Head Neck Surg.* **2015**, *14*, Doc04.
Magliocca, K.R.; Coker, N.A.; Parker, S.R. The head, neck, and systemic manifestations of levamisole-adulterated cocaine use. *J. Oral Maxillofac. Surg.* **2013**, *71*, 487–492. [CrossRef]
Magremanne, M.; Picheca, S.; Reychler, H. Etiologic diagnosis of jaw osteonecrosis, other than bisphosphonate and radiotherapy related osteonecrosis. *Rev. Stomatol. Chir. Maxillofac. Chir. Orale* **2014**, *115*, 45–50. [CrossRef]
Melo, C.A.A.; Guimarães, H.R.G.; Medeiros, R.C.F.; Souza, G.C.d.A.; dos Santos, P.B.D.; Tôrres, A.C.S.P. Oral changes in cocaine abusers: An integrative review. *Braz. J. Otorhinolaryngol.* **2022**, *88*, 633–641. [CrossRef]
Menick, F.J.; Salibian, A. Primary intranasal lining injury cause, deformities, and treatment plan. *Plast. Reconstr. Surg.* **2014**, *134*, 1045–1056. [CrossRef]

24. Molloy, E.S.; Langford, C.A. Vasculitis mimics. *Curr. Opin. Rheumatol.* **2008**, *20*, 29–34. [CrossRef] [PubMed]
25. Moreno-Artero, E.; Querol-Cisneros, E.; Rodríguez-Garijo, N.; Tomás-Velázquez, A.; Antoñanzas, J.; Secundino, F.; Gil-Sánc M.P.; España, A. Mucocutaneous manifestations of cocaine abuse: A review. *J. Eur. Acad. Dermatol. Venereol.* **2018**, *32*, 1420–1 [CrossRef]
26. Perper, J.A.; Van Thiel, D.H. Respiratory complications of cocaine abuse. In *Recent Developments in Alcoholism*; Springer: Bos MA, USA, 1992; Volume 10, pp. 363–377.
27. Rodrigo, J.P.; Suárez, C.; Rinaldo, A.; Devaney, K.O.; Carbone, A.; Barnes, L.; Heffner, D.K.; Ferlito, A. Idiopathic mid destructive disease: Fact or fiction. *Oral Oncol.* **2005**, *41*, 340–348. [CrossRef] [PubMed]
28. Sánchez-Puigdollers, A.; Just-Sarobé, M.; Pastor-Jané, L. Cutaneous and Mucosal Conditions Associated with Cocaine Use. *A Dermosifiliogr.* **2023**, *114*, 125–131. [CrossRef] [PubMed]
29. Sideris, G.; Davoutis, E.; Panagoulis, E.; Maragkoudakis, P.; Nikolopoulos, T.; Delides, A. A Systematic Review of Intracra Complications in Adults with Pott Puffy Tumor over Four Decades. *Brain Sci.* **2023**, *13*, 587. [CrossRef]
30. Silvestre, F.J.; Perez-Herbera, A.; Puente-Sandoval, A.; Bagán, J.V. Hard palate perforation in cocaine abusers: A systematic rev *Clin. Oral Investig.* **2010**, *14*, 621–628. [CrossRef]
31. Trimarchi, M.; Bertazzoni, G.; Bussi, M. Cocaine induced midline destructive lesions. *Rhinology* **2014**, *52*, 104–111. [CrossRef
32. Walker, A.; Joshi, A.; D'Souza, A. Care of the Cocaine User with Nasal Deformity. *Facial Plast. Surg.* **2017**, *33*, 411–418.
33. Palmero-Sánchez, B.; Faelens, G.; Corriols-Noval, P.; López-Simón, E.; Morales-Angulo, C. Manifestaciones de cabeza y cu secundarias al uso de cocaína. Revisión bibliográfica. *Rev. ORL* **2022**, *13*, 55–70.
34. Smith, J.C.; Kacker, A.; Anand, V.K. Midline nasal and hard palate destruction in cocaine abusers and cocaine's role in rhinol practice. *Ear Nose Throat J.* **2002**, *81*, 172–177. [CrossRef] [PubMed]
35. Marquez, J.; Aguirre, L.; Muñoz, C.; Echeverri, A.; Restrepo, M.; Pinto, L.F. Cocaine-Levamisole-Induced Vasculitis/Vasculopa Syndrome. *Curr. Rheumatol. Rep.* **2017**, *19*, 36. [CrossRef]
36. Pedro, B.; Meleiro, M.; Marinho, A. Not All ENT Granulomas Are Wegener's—Keep Tuberculosis in Mind. *Eur. J. Case Rep. Int Med.* **2020**, *7*, 001469. [PubMed]
37. Yaseen, K.; Nevares, A.; Tamaki, H. A Spotlight on Drug-Induced Vasculitis. *Curr. Rheumatol. Rep.* **2022**, *24*, 323–336. [Cross
38. Molteni, M.; Saibene, A.M.; Luciano, K.; Maccari, A. Snorting the clivus away: An extreme case of cocaine-induced mid destructive lesion. *BMJ Case Rep.* **2016**, *2016*, bcr2016216393. [CrossRef]
39. Taylor, A.; McLeod, G. Basic pharmacology of local anaesthetics. *BJA Educ.* **2020**, *20*, 34–41. [CrossRef] [PubMed]
40. Liao, B.S.; Hilsinger, R.L., Jr.; Rasgon, B.M.; Matsuoka, K.; Adour, K.K. A preliminary study of cocaine absorption from the n mucosa. *Laryngoscope* **1999**, *109*, 98–102. [CrossRef]
41. Ashchi, M.; Wiedemann, H.P.; James, K.B. Cardiac complication from use of cocaine and phenylephrine in nasal septoplasty. *A Otolaryngol. Head Neck Surg.* **1995**, *121*, 681–684. [CrossRef]
42. McGrath, J.; McGrath, A.; Burdett, J.; Shokri, T.; Cohn, J.E. Investigation of topical intranasal cocaine for sinonasal procedure randomized, phase III clinical trial. *Int. Forum Allergy Rhinol.* **2020**, *10*, 981–990. [CrossRef]
43. Becker, D.E.; Reed, K.L. Essentials of Local Anesthetic Pharmacology. *Anesth. Prog.* **2006**, *53*, 98–108. [CrossRef]
44. Lanzillotta, M.; Campochiaro, C.; Trimarchi, M.; Arrigoni, G.; Gerevini, S.; Milani, R.; Bozzolo, E.; Biafora, M.; Venturini Cicalese, M.P.; et al. Deconstructing IgG4-related disease involvement of midline structures: Comparison to common mimic *Mod. Rheumatol.* **2017**, *27*, 638–645. [CrossRef]
45. Eide, J.G.; Kshirsagar, R.S.; Birkenbeuel, J.L.; Abello, E.H.; Hobday, S.; Herzberg, S.; Wang, B.Y.; Palmer, J.N.; Adappa, N.D.; K E.C. Primary sinonasal lymphoma: A multi-institutional experience of clinical presentation, treatment, and outcomes. *Int. Fo Allergy Rhinol.* **2023**, *13*, 1492–1502. [CrossRef]
46. Wise, S.K.; Damask, C.; Roland, L.T.; Ebert, C.; Levy, J.M.; Lin, S.; Luong, A.; Rodriguez, K.; Sedaghat, A.R.; Toskala, E.; e International consensus statement on allergy and rhinology: Allergic rhinitis—2023. *Int. Forum Allergy Rhinol.* **2023**, *13*, 293–
47. Martinez, F.; Poet, T.S.; Pillai, R.; Erickson, J.; Estrada, A.L.; Watson, R.R. Cocaine metabolite (benzoylecgonine) in hair and u of drug users. *J. Anal. Toxicol.* **1993**, *17*, 138–142. [CrossRef] [PubMed]
48. Mahl, M.A.; Hirsch, M.; Sugg, U. Verification of the drug history given by potential blood donors: Results of drug screening combines hair and urine analysis. *Transfusion* **2000**, *40*, 637–641. [CrossRef]
49. Kim, J.A.; Ptolemy, A.S.; Melanson, S.E.F.; Janfaza, D.R.; Ross, E.L. The clinical impact of a false-positive urine cocaine scree result on a patient's pain management. *Pain. Med.* **2015**, *16*, 1073–1076. [CrossRef] [PubMed]
50. Shea, J.L. Bioanalytical methods for quantitation of levamisole, a widespread cocaine adulterant. *Clin. Chem. Lab. Med. (CC* **2013**, *51*, 205–212. [CrossRef] [PubMed]
51. Peyrière, H.; Léglise, Y.; Rousseau, A.; Cartier, C.; Gibaja, V.; Galland, P. Necrosis of the intranasal structures and soft palate result of heroin snorting: A case series. *Subst. Abus.* **2013**, *34*, 409–414. [CrossRef]

Cunningham, J.K.; Liu, L.-M.; Muramoto, M. Methamphetamine suppression and route of administration: Precursor regulation impacts on snorting, smoking, swallowing and injecting. *Addiction* **2008**, *103*, 1174–1186. [CrossRef]
Di Cosola, M.; Ambrosino, M.; Limongelli, L.; Favia, G.; Santarelli, A.; Cortelazzi, R.; Muzio, L.L. Cocaine-Induced Midline Destructive Lesions (CIMDL): A Real Challenge in Diagnosis. *Int. J. Environ. Res. Public Health* **2021**, *18*, 7831. [CrossRef]
Vocci, F.J.; Montoya, I.D. Psychological treatments for stimulant misuse, comparing and contrasting those for amphetamine dependence and those for cocaine dependence. *Curr. Opin. Psychiatry* **2009**, *22*, 263–268. [CrossRef] [PubMed]
Kampman, K.M. The treatment of cocaine use disorder. *Sci. Adv.* **2019**, *5*, eaax1532. [CrossRef] [PubMed]
Laroche, F.; Rostaing, S.; Aubrun, F.; Perrot, S. Pain management in heroin and cocaine users. *Jt. Bone Spine* **2012**, *79*, 446–450. [CrossRef] [PubMed]
Ortiz-Seller, A.; Hernández-Pons, A.; Pascual, E.V.; Pérez, A.C.; Gaitón, R.D.; Albert-Fort, M. Severe Cocaine-Induced Midline Destructive Lesions (CIMDL) Leading to Orbital Apex Syndrome and Peripheral Ulcerative Keratitis. *Ocul. Immunol. Inflamm.* **2022**, *30*, 1956–1960. [CrossRef]
Lascaratos, G.; McHugh, J.; McCarthy, K.; Bunting, H. Advanced cocaine-related necrotising sinusitis presenting with restrictive ophthalmolplegia. *Orbit* **2016**, *35*, 164–166. [CrossRef]
de Lange, T.E.; Simsek, S.; Kramer, M.H.H.; Nanayakkara, P.W.B. A case of cocaine-induced panhypopituitarism with human neutrophil elastase-specific anti-neutrophil cytoplasmic antibodies. *Eur. J. Endocrinol.* **2009**, *160*, 499–502. [CrossRef]
Brembilla, C.; Lanterna, L.A.; Risso, A.; Bombana, E.; Gritti, P.; Trezzi, R.; Bonaldi, G.; Biroli, F. Craniovertebral junction instability as an extension of cocaine-induced midline destructive lesions: Case report. *J. Neurosurg. Spine* **2015**, *23*, 159–165. [CrossRef]
Ciporen, J.; Lucke-Wold, B.; Gillham, H.; Cua, D.; Kim, J.; Akins, P. Paramedian forehead flap for repair of refractory high-flow anterior skull base CSF leak. *Turk. Neurosurg.* 2017; *online ahead of print*. [CrossRef]
Wang, W.; Vincent, A.; Shokri, T.; Hilger, P.; Ducic, Y. Septal Perforation Repair Using Bilateral Rotational Flaps With Interposed Mastoid Periosteal Graft. *Laryngoscope* **2021**, *131*, 1497–1500. [CrossRef]
Colletti, G.; Autelitano, L.; Chiapasco, M.; Biglioli, F.; Giovanditto, F.; Mandalà, M.; Allevi, F. Comprehensive surgical management of cocaine-induced midline destructive lesions. *J. Oral Maxillofac. Surg.* **2014**, *72*, 1395.e1–1395.e10. [CrossRef]
Colletti, G.; Allevi, F.; Valassina, D.; Bertossi, D.; Biglioli, F. Repair of cocaine-related oronasal fistula with forearm radial free flap. *J. Craniofac. Surg.* **2013**, *24*, 1734–1738. [CrossRef]
Hasin, D.S.; O'brien, C.P.; Auriacombe, M.; Borges, G.; Bucholz, K.; Budney, A.; Compton, W.M.; Crowley, T.; Ling, W.; Petry, N.M.; et al. DSM-5 Criteria for Substance Use Disorders: Recommendations and Rationale. *Am. J. Psychiatry* **2013**, *170*, 834–851. [CrossRef] [PubMed]
Germonpre, P.; Levie, P.; Dehalleux, C.; Caers, D. ENT indications for Hyperbaric Oxygen Therapy. *B-ENT* **2016**, *12* (Suppl. S26), 87–106.
Wells, E.A.; Peterson, P.L.; Gainey, R.R.; Hawkins, J.D.; Catalano, R.F. Outpatient treatment for cocaine abuse: A controlled comparison of relapse prevention and twelve-step approaches. *Am. J. Drug Alcohol. Abuse.* **1994**, *20*, 1–17. [CrossRef] [PubMed]
Weiss, R.D.; Griffin, M.L.; Najavits, L.M.; Hufford, C.; Kogan, J.; Thompson, H.J.; Albeck, J.H.; Bishop, S.; Daley, D.C.; Mercer, D.; et al. Self-help activities in cocaine dependent patients entering treatment: Results from NIDA collaborative cocaine treatment study. *Drug Alcohol. Depend.* **1996**, *43*, 79–86. [CrossRef]
Weiss, R.D.; Griffin, M.L.; Gallop, R.J.; Najavits, L.M.; Frank, A.; Crits-Christoph, P.; Thase, M.E.; Blaine, J.; Gastfriend, D.R.; Daley, D.; et al. The effect of 12-step self-help group attendance and participation on drug use outcomes among cocaine-dependent patients. *Drug Alcohol. Depend.* **2005**, *77*, 177–184. [CrossRef]
Fokkens, W.J.; Lund, V.J.; Hopkins, C.; Hellings, P.W.; Kern, R.; Reitsma, S.; Toppila-Salmi, S.; Bernal-Sprekelsen, M.; Mullol, J.; Alobid, I.; et al. European Position Paper on Rhinosinusitis and Nasal Polyps 2020. *Rhinology* **2020**, *58* (Suppl. S29), 1–464. [CrossRef]

Journal of
Personalized Medicine

MDPI

Article

Repurposing SGLT-2 Inhibitors as a Novel Therapeutic Strateg for Treatment-Resistant Meniere's Disease

Sun-Uk Lee [1,2] and Euyhyun Park [2,3,*]

1 Department of Neurology, Korea University College of Medicine, Seoul 02841, Republic of Korea; sulee716@gmail.com
2 Neurotology Laboratory, Korea University Anam Hospital, Seoul 02841, Republic of Korea
3 Department of Otorhinolaryngology-Head and Neck Surgery, Korea University College of Medicine, 73, Goryeodae-ro, Seongbuk-gu, Seoul 02841, Republic of Korea
* Correspondence: peath@naver.com or randoll@korea.ac.kr; Tel.: +82-2-920-6636

Abstract: Background: Meniere's disease (MD) is a chronic inner ear disorder affecting approximately 0.2% of the population, with 30% of patients remaining refractory to conventional treatments. The pathophysiology involves endolymphatic hydrops, suggesting that agents affecting fluid homeostasis might provide therapeutic benefit. Sodium-glucose cotransporter 2 (SGLT-2) inhibitors, originally developed for diabetes, offer unique mechanisms including natriuresis and osmotic diuresis that may address the underlying fluid imbalance in MD. **Methods**: We conducted a retrospective observational study at the Korea University Anam Hospital, analyzing the medical records of patients with definite MD (Bárány Society criteria) who received off-label empagliflozin 10 mg daily between January 2023 and December 2023. Six patients (3 men, 3 women; mean age 55.8 years) with treatment-resistant MD were identified who had failed conventional therapy for at least 3 months. Primary outcomes included changes in pure tone threshold average (PTA), low-frequency threshold average (LFA), vertigo episode frequency, and vertigo severity using visual analog scale (VAS) scores, assessed at baseline and after 3 months of treatment. **Results:** All patients demonstrated clinically significant improvements in both auditory and vestibular symptoms. Mean PTA improved from 31.4 dB to 20.8 dB (improvement of 10.6 dB, $p < 0.05$). Low-frequency hearing showed more substantial recovery, with LFA improving from 37.2 dB to 15.6 dB (improvement of 21.6 dB, $p < 0.01$). Vertigo frequency decreased dramatically from 1.6 episodes per month to 0.1 episodes per month, with four patients experiencing a complete resolution of vertigo episodes. VAS scores for vertigo severity decreased from 5.2 to 0.5. Treatment was well-tolerated, with only minor adverse effects reported in two patients: transient polyuria in one patient and 5 kg weight loss in another, both consistent with the known pharmacological profile of SGLT-2 inhibitors. **Conclusions**: This preliminary study suggests a potential clinical benefit of repurposing SGLT-2 inhibitors for treatment-resistant MD. However, the retrospective design and inherent limitations prevent definitive conclusions about causality. The significant improvements observed in both hearing thresholds and vestibular symptoms warrant further investigation through randomized controlled trials with objective outcome measures to establish the true efficacy of this therapeutic approach.

Keywords: Meniere's disease; SGLT-2 inhibitors; drug repurposing; endolymphatic hydrops; personalized medicine; treatment-resistant

1. Introduction

Meniere's disease (MD) is a chronic inner ear disorder characterized by episodic vertigo, fluctuating sensorineural hearing loss, tinnitus, and aural fullness [1]. With a prevalence of approximately 0.2% globally [2], MD typically manifests in middle age and represents a significant cause of disability due to unpredictable vertigo attacks that severely impact quality of life and employment [3].

The pathophysiology of MD centers on endolymphatic hydrops, an excessive accumulation of endolymph within inner ear compartments, first histologically demonstrated by Hallpike and Cairns in 1938 [4]. Modern gadolinium-enhanced magnetic resonance imaging has enabled the in vivo visualization of endolymphatic hydrops, confirming its presence in most MD patients [5]. Recent research has revealed MD as a complex multifactorial disease involving genetic, immunological, and environmental factors, with distinct inflammatory signatures including elevated pro-inflammatory cytokines [6,7].

Current management follows a stepwise approach, beginning with lifestyle modifications and conservative treatments. First-line therapies include dietary sodium restriction, diuretics, and betahistine [8]. However, evidence for conventional treatments remains limited, with systematic reviews highlighting insufficient high-quality data [9]. The landmark BEMED trial failed to demonstrate the significant benefits of betahistine over placebo [10], and meta-analyses showed only modest evidence for diuretic efficacy [11]. Despite these approaches, approximately 30% of patients fail to respond adequately to conventional treatment, highlighting the urgent need for novel therapeutic strategies [12].

Sodium-glucose cotransporter 2 (SGLT-2) inhibitors represent a promising therapeutic candidate for MD through several mechanisms relevant to inner ear pathophysiology. These agents work by selectively inhibiting SGLT-2 receptors in the kidney, blocking glucose reabsorption and leading to glucosuria with natriuresis and osmotic diuresis [13]. Beyond glucose lowering, SGLT-2 inhibitors demonstrate pleiotropic effects including the following: (1) gradual and sustained volume reduction through physiological diuresis, potentially providing more stable inner ear fluid homeostasis compared to traditional diuretics; (2) anti-inflammatory properties, reducing circulating pro-inflammatory cytokines that may contribute to MD pathogenesis; and (3) microvascular improvements through enhanced endothelial function [14,15].

The drug repurposing approach offers significant advantages for rare conditions like refractory MD, with established safety profiles potentially accelerating clinical evaluation [16]. While a recent preclinical study found empagliflozin ineffective in preventing hydrops development in mice, their study focused on prevention rather than treatment of the established disease, and clinical translation remains to be determined [17].

To our knowledge, this represents the first clinical investigation exploring SGLT-2 inhibitor repurposing for established MD treatment in humans. This retrospective analysis examines clinical outcomes in patients who received off-label SGLT-2 inhibitor therapy after failing conventional treatment, providing preliminary evidence to inform future prospective trials.

2. Methods

2.1. Study Design and Participants

This retrospective study was conducted using clinical data from patients treated at the Neuroscience Center, under the approval of the Institutional Review Board of Korea University Anam Hospital (IRB No. 2023AN0297, approval date: 10 July 2023). The IRB approval was part of a broader institutional registry protocol. A continuing review approval was obtained on 20 June 2024. Medical records were reviewed for patients with definite MD according to the Bárány Society criteria who received off-label SGLT-2 inhibitor treatment between January 2023 and December 2023 [18].

Six patients (3 men, 3 women) with definite MD were identified who had documented failure to respond to conventional treatment, defined as persistent symptoms despite at least 3 months of standard treatment approaches, including diuretics and/or betahistine. These patients were subsequently prescribed off-label empagliflozin based on clinical judgment considering the theoretical mechanism of action and refractory nature of their condition. None of the patients had diabetes mellitus, metabolic syndrome, chronic kidney disease, or heart failure at the time of treatment initiation. Baseline clinical characteristics of the patients are presented in Table 1.

Table 1. Baseline characteristics of patients with refractory Meniere's disease.

Patient	Age/Sex	Disease Duration (Months)	Affected Ear	Previous Treatment	Duration of Previous Treatment (Months)
1	45/M	12	Right	HCTZ 25 mg QD + Amiloride 5 mg QD + Betahistine 24 mg BID	6
2	67/F	6	Right	HCTZ 25 mg QD + Amiloride 5 mg QD + Betahistine 24 mg BID	3
3	65/F	12	Right	HCTZ 25 mg QD + Betahistine 24 mg BID	7
4	39/F	14	Right	HCTZ 25 mg QD + Betahistine 24 mg BID	6
5	56/M	19	Left	HCTZ 25 mg QD + Amiloride 5 mg QD + Betahistine 24 mg BID	6
6	63/M	10	Left	Isosorbide mononitrate 10 mL BID	10

Abbreviations: HCTZ, hydrochlorothiazide; QD, once daily; BID, twice daily.

2.2. Treatment Protocol

Patients with definite MD who had documented failure to respond to conventional treatment were transitioned directly to empagliflozin 10 mg orally once daily without a formal washout period. This approach was chosen to prevent potential symptom exacerbation during treatment interruption in these refractory patients. Vestibular suppressants (dimenhydrinate 50 mg or meclizine 25 mg) were permitted as rescue medication for acute vertigo episodes as needed.

2.3. Data Collection and Outcome Measures

Medical records were systematically reviewed to extract data on the following:

Primary outcome measures:

1. Change in pure tone threshold average (PTA), calculated as the average of thresholds at 0.5, 1, 2, and 4 kHz using the formula: (0.5 kHz + 2 × 1 kHz + 2 × 2 kHz + 4 kHz)/6.
2. Change in low-frequency threshold average (LFA), calculated as the average of thresholds at 0.25, 0.5, and 1 kHz.
3. Change in the frequency of definitive vertigo episodes per month.
4. Change in vertigo severity using a visual analog scale (VAS) consisting of a 100 mm horizontal line with anchor points of 0 ('no vertigo symptoms') and 10 ('worst possible vertigo symptoms'). Patients were instructed to mark their average symptom severity without numerical reference points visible.

5. Treatment-related adverse effects.

Assessments were performed at baseline and after 3 months of treatment based on available clinical records.

2.4. Statistical Analysis

Given the small sample size (n = 6), descriptive statistics were calculated for outcome measures. Pre- and post-treatment comparisons were performed using the Wilcoxon signed-rank test for paired non-parametric data, as normality could not be assumed with the small sample size. Statistical significance was set at $p < 0.05$. All statistical analyses were performed using SPSS version 28.0 (IBM Corp, Armonk, NY, USA). We acknowledge that the limited sample size substantially reduces statistical power and increases the risk of both type I and type II errors.

3. Results

3.1. Efficacy Outcomes

All patients demonstrated significant improvements in hearing thresholds and vertigo symptoms after 3 months of SGLT-2 inhibitor therapy. Mean PTA improved from 31.4 dB to 20.8 dB (improvement of 10.6 dB, $p < 0.05$). Low-frequency hearing showed more substantial recovery, with LFA improving from 37.2 dB to 15.6 dB (an improvement of 21.6 dB, $p < 0.01$). Vertigo frequency decreased dramatically from 1.6 episodes per month to 0.1 episodes per month, with four patients experiencing a complete resolution of vertigo episodes. VAS scores for vertigo severity decreased from 5.2 to 0.5. Detailed outcomes are presented in Table 2.

Table 2. Changes in hearing thresholds and vertigo parameters after 3 months of SGLT-2 inhibitor treatment.

arameter	Baseline	After 3 Months	Mean Change
ure-tone average, dB *	31.4 (15.0–45.0)	20.8 (4.2–40.8)	−10.6
ow-frequency average, dB †	37.2 (16.7–55.0)	15.6 (5.0–28.3)	−21.6
ertigo episodes per month	1.6 (1.0–3.3)	0.1 (0–0.3)	−1.5
ertigo severity (VAS score, 0–10)	5.2 (3–7)	0.5 (0–2)	−4.7

* Pure-tone average was calculated as the average of thresholds at 0.5, 1, 2, and 4 kHz using the formula: (0.5 kHz + 2 × 1 kHz + 2 × 2 kHz + 4 kHz)/6. † Low-frequency average was calculated as the average of thresholds at 0.25, 0.5, and 1 kHz. Data are presented as mean (range). Abbreviation: VAS, visual analog scale.

The improvement in LFA was particularly notable, with a mean reduction of 21.6 dB, which is clinically significant for patients with Meniere's disease who typically experience greater hearing loss in the low frequencies. Four of the six patients experienced a complete resolution of vertigo episodes.

3.2. Safety Outcomes

Overall, SGLT-2 inhibitor therapy was well-tolerated. One patient experienced mild polyuria during the first week of treatment, which resolved spontaneously without intervention. Another patient experienced a 5 kg weight loss over the 3-month treatment period, which is consistent with the known effects of SGLT-2 inhibitors. No episodes of hypoglycemia, urinary tract infections, or genital infections were reported. All patients completed the full course of treatment with 100% adherence.

4. Discussion

This retrospective analysis suggests that repurposing SGLT-2 inhibitors may be effective in improving both auditory and vestibular symptoms in patients with MD who are refractory to conventional treatment. Patients showed robust improvement in vertigo frequency and hearing thresholds, with the complete resolution of vertigo episodes in four of six patients.

The beneficial effects of SGLT-2 inhibition may be attributed to several mechanisms. SGLT-2 inhibitors induce natriuresis and osmotic diuresis, which could reduce systemic fluid volume and, consequently, endolymphatic pressure [19]. Unlike traditional diuretics, SGLT-2 inhibitors promote more gradual and sustained volume reduction, potentially providing more stable fluid homeostasis [20]. This physiological approach to diuresis may be particularly advantageous in MD, where sudden changes in fluid balance could potentially exacerbate symptoms. Additionally, SGLT-2 inhibitors have demonstrated pleiotropic effects, including improvements in vascular function and reduction in oxidative stress, which may address microvascular hypoperfusion as a potential pathomechanism of MD [21].

Recent advances in understanding inner ear physiology have revealed the presence of glucose transporters in cochlear and vestibular tissues. The inner ear's glucose metabolism is critical for maintaining cellular energy homeostasis, particularly in hair cells and supporting cells that are metabolically active [22]. SGLT-2 inhibitors may influence inner ear glucose handling and fluid balance through both direct effects on local glucose transporters and indirect effects via systemic metabolic changes. The reduction in systemic glucose levels and associated osmotic effects may contribute to decreased endolymphatic volume and pressure.

The anti-inflammatory properties of SGLT-2 inhibitors represent another potential therapeutic mechanism. Recent research has identified inflammatory processes as key contributors to MD pathogenesis, with elevated levels of pro-inflammatory cytokines found in MD patients [6,7]. SGLT-2 inhibitors have been shown to reduce circulating inflammatory markers, potentially addressing the inflammatory component of MD pathophysiology.

The improvement in the low-frequency hearing thresholds is particularly significant, as these frequencies are typically most affected in MD [23]. This finding suggests that SGLT-2 inhibition may address the underlying pathophysiology of endolymphatic hydrops rather than simply masking symptoms. The preferential improvement in low-frequency hearing aligns with the expected effects of reducing endolymphatic pressure, as low-frequency hearing is most sensitive to changes in inner ear fluid dynamics [24].

Traditional diuretics used in MD management primarily target the distal convoluted tubule and collecting duct, and can cause electrolyte imbalances with inconsistent effects on endolymphatic homeostasis [25]. In contrast, SGLT-2 inhibitors offer a more physiological approach to diuresis by blocking glucose reabsorption in the proximal tubule, leading to glucosuria-induced osmotic diuresis [26]. This mechanism may provide more consistent fluid balance effects compared to traditional diuretics, potentially explaining the dramatic reduction in vertigo episodes observed in our patients.

The concept of personalized medicine in MD management is gaining recognition, with acknowledgment that different patients may respond to different therapeutic approaches based on their underlying pathophysiology [27]. Patients with predominantly fluid retention-related symptoms may be ideal candidates for SGLT-2 inhibitor therapy, particularly those with comorbid metabolic conditions. Future research should focus on identifying biomarkers or clinical characteristics that can predict the response to SGLT-2 inhibitor therapy, enabling more targeted treatment approaches.

The drug repurposing approach offers several advantages in addressing unmet medical needs in rare conditions like refractory MD. SGLT-2 inhibitors have well-established safety profiles from extensive use in diabetes management, potentially accelerating their evaluation for alternative indications [28]. Moreover, the existing clinical experience provides valuable insights into safety profiles, drug interactions, and contraindications. The cost-effectiveness of repurposing existing medications compared to developing novel therapies represents another significant advantage, particularly important for rare conditions where pharmaceutical investment may be limited. The excellent tolerability profile observed in our study is consistent with the known safety characteristics of SGLT-2 inhibitors. The mild adverse effects, including transient polyuria and modest weight loss, are generally manageable and may even provide additional benefits for patients with comorbid conditions such as hypertension or obesity. This tolerability advantage over traditional treatments may improve patient adherence and long-term treatment outcomes.

This study has several important limitations that must be acknowledged. First, the retrospective observational design without a control group fundamentally limits our ability to establish causality between SGLT-2 inhibitor treatment and clinical improvements. The natural fluctuating course of MD makes it particularly challenging to distinguish treatment effects from natural disease progression or placebo effects. Second, the absence of objective measures such as gadolinium-enhanced MRI to assess endolymphatic hydrops represents a critical limitation [5,29]. Third, the small sample size (n = 6) and relatively short follow-up period (3 months) limit the generalizability of findings and prevent the assessment of long-term treatment sustainability. Fourth, the lack of a formal washout period means that potential residual effects from previous treatments cannot be completely excluded. Fifth, the discordance with preclinical findings by Pålbrink et al., who found empagliflozin ineffective in preventing endolymphatic hydrops in a mouse model, raises questions about mechanism and translational relevance, though their study focused on prevention rather than treatment of the established disease.

Future research should prioritize randomized controlled trials with adequate sample sizes and appropriate control groups to establish definitive efficacy and safety profiles. Studies should incorporate objective outcome measures, including gadolinium-enhanced MRI assessment of endolymphatic hydrops, vestibular function testing, and validated quality of life instruments. Long-term follow-up studies are essential to determine treatment durability and identify potential late adverse effects.

The investigation of optimal dosing regimens, treatment duration, and patient selection criteria for SGLT-2 inhibitor therapy in MD represents another critical research priority. Pharmacokinetic studies examining the penetration of these agents into inner ear fluids would provide valuable mechanistic insights. Additionally, combination therapy approaches utilizing SGLT-2 inhibitors with other treatments may offer synergistic benefits and should be explored.

The development of biomarkers to predict treatment response would significantly advance personalized medicine approaches in MD management. This could include genetic markers, inflammatory profiles, or metabolic parameters that identify the patients most likely to benefit from SGLT-2 inhibitor therapy.

Despite these limitations, our findings provide compelling preliminary evidence supporting the potential repurposing of SGLT-2 inhibitors as a therapeutic candidate in treatment-resistant MD, warranting further investigation through properly designed clinical trials.

5. Conclusions

This preliminary retrospective study suggests that SGLT-2 inhibitor therapy may have potential benefits for patients with treatment-resistant MD. However, the observational design and inherent limitations prevent definitive conclusions about causality. The significant improvements observed in both hearing thresholds and vestibular symptoms warrant further investigation through properly designed randomized controlled trials with objective outcome measures, including gadolinium-enhanced MRI assessment of endolymphatic hydrops, to establish the true efficacy of this therapeutic approach.

Author Contributions: Concept and Design: E.P.; Supervision and Critical Review: S.-U.L.; Data Collection and Processing: S.-U.L. and E.P.; Analysis and Interpretation: E.P.; Literature Search: S.-U.L. and E.P.; Manuscript Writing: S.-U.L. and E.P. All authors have read and agreed to the published version of the manuscript.

Funding: This research was supported by the Basic Science Research Program through the National Research Foundation of Korea (NRF) funded by the Ministry of Education (NRF-2021R1I1A1A01052753) and the Ministry of Science and ICT (2022R1A4A1018869). These funding sources provided only financial support and played no specific scientific role in this study.

Institutional Review Board Statement: This study was conducted in accordance with the Declaration of Helsinki, and approved by the Institutional Review Board of Korea University Anam Hospital (IRB No. 2023AN0297, approval date: 10 July 2023; renewal date: 20 June 2024).

Informed Consent Statement: Informed consent was obtained from all subjects involved in the study.

Data Availability Statement: The data that support the findings of this study are available from the corresponding author upon reasonable request. Due to privacy and ethical considerations, certain restrictions may apply to the availability of data.

Conflicts of Interest: The authors declare no conflict of interest.

References

1. Nakashima, T.; Pyykkö, I.; Arroll, M.A.; Casselbrant, M.L.; Foster, C.A.; Manzoor, N.F.; Megerian, C.A.; Naganawa, S.; Young, Y Meniere's disease. *Nat. Rev. Dis. Primers* **2016**, *2*, 16028. [CrossRef] [PubMed]
2. Alexander, T.H.; Harris, J.P. Current epidemiology of Meniere's syndrome. *Otolaryngol. Clin. N. Am.* **2010**, *43*, 965–970. [Cross
3. Tyrrell, J.; Whinney, D.J.; Ukoumunne, O.C.; Fleming, L.E.; Osborne, N.J. Prevalence, associated factors, and comorbid conditi for Meniere's disease. *Ear Hear.* **2014**, *35*, e162–e169. [CrossRef]
4. Hallpike, C.S.; Cairns, H. Observations on the pathology of Meniere's syndrome. *J. Laryngol. Otol.* **1938**, *53*, 625–655. [Cross
5. Naganawa, S.; Nakashima, T. Visualization of endolymphatic hydrops with MR imaging in patients with Meniere's disease related pathologies: Current status of its methods and clinical significance. *Jpn. J. Radiol.* **2014**, *32*, 191–204. [CrossRef]
6. Gazquez, I.; Soto-Varela, A.; Aran, I.; Santos, S.; Batuecas, A.; Trinidad, G.; Perez-Garrigues, H.; Gonzalez-Oller, C.; Acosta Lopez-Escamez, J.A. High prevalence of systemic autoimmune diseases in patients with Meniere's disease. *PLoS ONE* **201** e26759. [CrossRef]
7. Huang, C.; Wang, Q.; Pan, X.; Li, W.; Liu, W.; Jiang, W.; Huang, L.; Peng, A.; Zhang, Z. Up-Regulated Expression of Interfe Gamma, Interleukin-6 and Tumor Necrosis Factor-Alpha in the Endolymphatic Sac of Ménière's Disease Suggesting the L Inflammatory Response Underlies the Mechanism of This Disease. *Front. Neurol.* **2022**, *13*, 781031. [CrossRef]
8. Basura, G.J.; Adams, M.E.; Monfared, A.; Schwartz, S.R.; Antonelli, P.J.; Burkard, R.; Bush, M.L.; Bykowski, J.; Colandrea, Derebery, J.; et al. Clinical practice guideline: Meniere's disease. *Otolaryngol. Head Neck Surg.* **2020**, *162* (Suppl. 2), S1– [CrossRef]
9. van Esch, B.F.; van der Zaag-Loonen, H.; Bruintjes, T.D.; van Benthem, P.P.G. Betahistine in Ménière's Disease or Syndrome Systematic Review. *Audiol. Neurootol.* **2022**, *27*, 1–33. [CrossRef]
10. Adrion, C.; Fischer, C.S.; Wagner, J.; Gürkov, R.; Mansmann, U.; Strupp, M. Efficacy and safety of betahistine treatment in patie with Meniere's disease: Primary results of a long term, multicentre, double blind, randomised, placebo controlled, dose defin trial (BEMED trial). *BMJ* **2016**, *352*, h6816. [CrossRef] [PubMed]

Crowson, M.G.; Patki, A.; Tucci, D.L. A Systematic Review of Diuretics in the Medical Management of Ménière's Disease. *Otolaryngol. Head Neck Surg.* **2016**, *154*, 824–834. [CrossRef]
El Shafei, R.R.; Qotb, M. Comparison of the Effect of Three Treatment Interventions for the Control of Ménière's Disease: A Randomized Control Trial. *Egypt. J. Otolaryngol.* **2020**, *36*, 22. [CrossRef]
Abdul-Ghani, M.A.; Norton, L.; DeFronzo, R.A. Role of sodium-glucose cotransporter 2 (SGLT 2) inhibitors in the treatment of type 2 diabetes. *Endocr. Rev.* **2011**, *32*, 515–531. [CrossRef]
Salvatore, T.; Galiero, R.; Caturano, A.; Rinaldi, L.; Di Martino, A.; Albanese, G.; Di Salvo, J.; Epifani, R.; Marfella, R.; Docimo, G.; et al. An overview of the cardiorenal protective mechanisms of SGLT2 inhibitors. *Int. J. Mol. Sci.* **2022**, *23*, 3651. [CrossRef]
Bonnet, F.; Scheen, A.J. Effects of SGLT2 inhibitors on systemic and tissue low-grade inflammation: The potential contribution to diabetes complications and cardiovascular disease. *Diabetes Metab.* **2018**, *44*, 457–464. [CrossRef] [PubMed]
Pushpakom, S.; Iorio, F.; Eyers, P.A.; Escott, K.J.; Hopper, S.; Wells, A.; Doig, A.; Guilliams, T.; Latimer, J.; McNamee, C.; et al. Drug repurposing: Progress, challenges and recommendations. *Nat. Rev. Drug Discov.* **2019**, *18*, 41–58. [CrossRef] [PubMed]
Pålbrink, A.K.; In 't Zandt, R.; Magnusson, M.; Degerman, E. Empagliflozin does not prevent endolymphatic hydrops development in a mouse model. *Acta Otolaryngol.* **2023**, *143*, 127–133. [CrossRef]
Lopez-Escamez, J.A.; Carey, J.; Chung, W.H.; Goebel, J.A.; Magnusson, M.; Mandalà, M.; Newman-Toker, D.E.; Strupp, M.; Suzuki, M.; Trabalzini, F.; et al. Diagnostic criteria for Menière's disease. *J. Vestib. Res.* **2015**, *25*, 1–7. [CrossRef]
Vallon, V.; Thomson, S.C. Targeting renal glucose reabsorption to treat hyperglycaemia: The pleiotropic effects of SGLT2 inhibition. *Diabetologia* **2017**, *60*, 215–225. [CrossRef] [PubMed]
Cherney, D.Z.; Perkins, B.A.; Soleymanlou, N.; Maione, M.; Lai, V.; Lee, A.; Fagan, N.M.; Woerle, H.J. Johansen, O.E.; Broedl, U.C.; et al. Renal hemodynamic effect of sodium-glucose cotransporter 2 inhibition in patients with type 1 diabetes mellitus. *Circulation* **2014**, *129*, 587–597. [CrossRef]
Packer, M. Mechanisms leading to differential hypotensive effects of sodium-glucose cotransporter 2 inhibitors in experimental hypertension. *Cardiovasc. Diabetol.* **2018**, *17*, 24.
Spicer, S.S.; Schulte, B.A. The fine structure of spiral ligament cells relates to ion return to the stria and varies with place-frequency. *Hear. Res.* **1996**, *100*, 80–100. [CrossRef] [PubMed]
Yamakawa, K. Low-frequency sensorineural hearing loss in Meniere's disease. *Otolaryngol. Head. Neck Surg.* **1997**, *117*, 555–561.
Schaette, R.; McAlpine, D. Tinnitus with a normal audiogram: Physiological evidence for hidden hearing loss and computational model. *J. Neurosci.* **2011**, *31*, 13452–13457. [CrossRef]
Hain, T.C.; Uddin, M. Pharmacological treatment of vertigo. *CNS Drugs* **2003**, *17*, 85–100. [CrossRef]
Heerspink, H.J.L.; Perkins, B.A.; Fitchett, D.H.; Husain, M.; Cherney, D.Z. Sodium glucose cotransporter 2 inhibitors in the treatment of diabetes mellitus: Cardiovascular and kidney effects, potential mechanisms, and clinical applications. *Circulation* **2016**, *134*, 752–772. [CrossRef]
Espinosa-Sanchez, J.M.; Lopez-Escamez, J.A. Menière's disease. *Handb. Clin. Neurol.* **2016**, *137*, 257–277. [PubMed]
Nosengo, N. Can. you teach old drugs new tricks? *Nature* **2016**, *534*, 314–316. [CrossRef]
Pyykkö, I.; Nakashima, T.; Yoshida, T.; Zou, J.; Naganawa, S. Meniere's disease: A reappraisal supported by a variable latency of symptoms and the MRI visualisation of endolymphatic hydrops. *BMJ Open* **2013**, *3*, e001555. [CrossRef]

Journal of
Personalized Medicine

MDPI

Article

Transoral Cordectomy with Microelectrodes (TOMES) on an Outpatient Basis: Advancing Patient Comfort and Personalized Care Through Predictive Models

Cristina Rodríguez-Prado [1], Natsuki Oishi [1,2,*], Ernesto Fernández-Vidal [1], José Ramón Alba-García [1] and Enrique Zapater [1,2]

1 ENT Department, Valencia University General Hospital, 46014 Valencia, Spain; rodriguez_cripra@gva.es (C.R.-P.); ernestofernandez@bellvitgehospital.cat (E.F.-V.); alba_josgar@gva.es (J.R.A.-G.); enrique.zapater@uv.es (E.Z.)
2 Faculty of Medicine and Odontology, Valencia University, 46010 Valencia, Spain
* Correspondence: miriam.n.oishi@uv.es

Abstract: Background/Objectives: Outpatient surgery enhances patient comfort while reduces surgical wait times and healthcare costs compared to inpatient procedures. This study evaluates the individual feasibility of performing transoral trans muscular cordectomies with microelectrodes (TOMES) on an outpatient basis. **Methods**: This observational study analyses TOMES types III, IV, and V cordectomies performed from January 2002 to December 2023. Key metrics include patient demographics, procedural details, incidence of bleeding, anticoagulation and other comorbidities. **Results**: Of the 143 procedures, 127 were cancer-related, while 16 were due to bilateral vocal cord paralysis. The average age was 65, with a predominantly male cohort (92%). Postoperative hemorrhage occurred in four cases, primarily among oncological patients, but there was no correlation with anticoagulation therapy. A personalized predictive model for bleeding risk was developed based on patient-specific characteristics and observed outcomes. Additionally, performing the procedure on an outpatient basis decreased healthcare costs and wait times for patients with T1/T2 glottic carcinoma. **Conclusions**: The findings indicate that TOMES type III or higher cordectomies can be safely performed on an outpatient basis, through the use of a personalized predictive model for each case and with appropriate postoperative monitoring. This approach has the potential to lower healthcare costs and improve patient quality of life through individualized assessments and structured risk analysis.

Keywords: cordectomy; laryngeal cancer; microelectrode; quality of life; healthcare costs; individual predictive model

1. Introduction

Laryngeal cancer represents approximately one-third of all head and neck malignancies, with a reported 5-year overall survival rate ranging from 50% to 60% [1]. It remains a significant cause of morbidity and mortality worldwide. Among laryngeal tumours, the glottic region is the most commonly affected site, accounting for nearly half of the cases, although this proportion may vary depending on the population and geographical region studied [2]. The widespread use of advanced diagnostic tools such as high-definition videolaryngoscopy and narrow-band imaging has facilitated the earlier detection of glottic carcinomas. Consequently, an increasing number of cases are now diagnosed at early clinical stages (T1–T2), allowing for less invasive and organ-preserving treatment approaches [3]. For early stage glottic cancer, both transoral surgery and radiotherapy are considered standard treatment options. While some studies suggest that surgical intervention may offer better local control, faster recovery, and lower treatment-associated morbidity, other analyses report no statistically significant differences in oncologic outcomes between the two modalities [3,4]. However, surgery has been shown in some contexts to offer a more favourable cost-effectiveness profile compared to radiotherapy [5].

Among the surgical approaches, transoral microelectrode surgery (TOMES) has emerged as a reliable alternative to laser microlaryngoscopy. TOMES enables precise dissection with simultaneous coagulation, preserves tactile feedback, reduces operative time, and is significantly more cost-efficient than CO_2 laser systems [6,7].

In these cases of T1/T2 glottic tumours, the indicated surgical procedure is the cordectomy, which consists of the partial or complete excision of the vocal fold, typically performed for oncological or functional indications. The extent and depth of resection is classified according to the system proposed by the European Laryngological Society (ELS) [8,9], which provides a standardized framework for endoscopic cordectomy procedures. This classification is based on anatomical criteria and distinguishes between six main types (Figure 1):

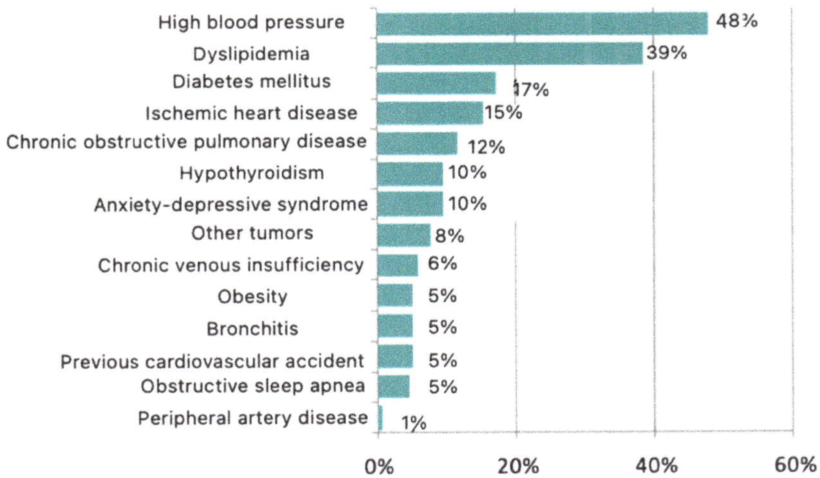

Figure 1. Concomitant diseases of the patients under study.

Type I: Subepithelial cordectomy
Type II: Subligamental cordectomy
Type III: Transmuscular cordectomy
Type IV: Total cordectomy
Type V: Extended cordectomy
Type VI: Cordectomy involving the anterior commissure

Furthermore, type V cordectomies are subdivided depending on the anatomical structures involved:

Va: Extension to the contralateral vocal fold including the anterior commissure
Vb: Involvement of the arytenoid
Vc: Extension into the subglottic space
Vd: Involvement of the laryngeal ventricle

This classification allows surgeons to plan the extent of resection with greater precision based on tumour size, location, and infiltration depth, and it facilitates comparison of surgical outcomes across centres. Type III, IV, and V cordectomies entail deeper tissue resection and carry a higher theoretical risk of postoperative complications such as bleeding or prolonged hospitalization. Assessing these more complex procedures is crucial to determine the safety and feasibility of implementing outpatient protocols for selected patients.

In our institution, TOMES has been the standard technique for performing cordectomies for over two decades, consistently yielding excellent oncological outcomes with minimal postoperative complications. This experience has fostered the expansion of TOMES procedures into the outpatient setting.

In parallel, there has been a growing global trend toward ambulatory surgery across multiple specialties. In addition, medicine is increasingly being practised in a more personalized way, with each case being assessed individually and treatment always adapted to the situation and condition of each patient at any given time.

Ambulatory surgical models tailored to each person offer numerous benefits, including enhanced patient satisfaction, reduced hospital-acquired complications, and faster return to daily activities [10]. From a health systems perspective, same-day discharge protocols reduce healthcare expenditures and optimize surgical wait times by improving the turnover of operating room resources [11,12].

In this context, assessing the safety and individual feasibility of performing more extensive cordectomies for glottic tumours in an outpatient setting is of growing clinical relevance. Understanding the predictors of postoperative complications, particularly bleeding and prolonged hospitalization, is essential to refine patient selection criteria and ensure optimal perioperative outcomes.

The primary objective of this study is to analyze the individual risk factors associated with postoperative complications, particularly bleeding and prolonged hospital stay, in patients undergoing transmuscular or extended cordectomies (types III, IV, and V) using transoral microelectrode surgery (TOMES).

Based on this analysis, we aim to develop personalized predictive models that can estimate the likelihood of successful outpatient management for each patient. The ultimate goal is to support clinical decision-making regarding ambulatory surgery eligibility, with the intention of enhancing patient comfort and quality of life, optimizing hospital resource allocation, reducing surgical waiting times, and lowering overall healthcare costs.

2. Materials and Methods

A retrospective observational study was conducted at a single tertiary care centre, based on the review of medical records from patients who underwent transoral microelectrode surgery (TOMES) for transmuscular (type III) or extended (types IV and V) cordectomies between January 2002 and December 2023 [8,9].

Eligible patients were those who underwent type III, IV, or V cordectomies using TOMES and fulfilled all protocol-defined criteria. Exclusion criteria included intraoperative conversion to open surgery, the use of alternative surgical instrumentation, or any deviation from standard surgical indications. Furthermore, type I and II cordectomies were excluded, as these are currently performed on an outpatient basis at our institution.

Based on epidemiological data from the Spanish Network of Cancer Registries (REDECAN 2025), the overall incidence of laryngeal cancer in Spain is estimated at 6.1 cases per 100,000 inhabitants per year when both sexes are considered. Approximately 60% of laryngeal cancers originate in the glottis, and two-thirds of glottic carcinomas are diagnosed at an early stage. In our healthcare area, which serves a population of approximately 390,000 inhabitants, the expected incidence of early-stage (T1–T2) glottic squamous cell carcinoma was therefore estimated at 2.5 cases per 100,000 person-years, corresponding to 9–10 new cases annually.

Assuming a Poisson distribution for rare events, the required sample size was calculated to achieve a 95% confidence interval with a predefined relative precision. The number of cases was derived using the formula: $k \approx (r \times 1.96)^2$ where k represents the required number of cases and r the desired relative margin of error.

To estimate the incidence with a relative precision of ±20%, a minimum of approximately 96 cases was required. Based on the expected annual incidence within our reference population, the accrual period was planned accordingly to meet this requirement.

Out of 151 cordectomies initially performed with TOMES, 8 cases were excluded due to conversion to open surgery. Thus, a total of 143 cordectomies met the inclusion criteria and were included in the final analysis.

Baseline variables included sex, age, underlying pathology (glottic carcinoma or vocal cord paralysis), and risk factors such as smoking and alcohol use. Comorbidities were recorded, including arterial hypertension, dyslipidemia, ischemic heart disease, diabetes mellitus, chronic obstructive pulmonary disease (COPD), hypothyroidism, anxiety-depressive disorder, malignancy at another site, chronic venous insufficiency, obesity, chronic bronchitis, prior cerebrovascular accident, obstructive sleep apnoea, and peripheral arterial disease. Surgical data encompassed the type of cordectomy and anticoagulant use on the day of surgery. Oral anticoagulants (including vitamin K antagonists, direct thrombin inhibitors, and factor Xa inhibitors) were discontinued 48 to 72 h before surgery following hematology department recommendations. Bridging therapy with low-molecular-weight heparin (LMWH) was initiated and maintained until 24 to 48 h after the procedure, provided no adverse events occurred. Oral anticoagulation was then reintroduced according to clinical stability and standard protocol. Postoperative variables included the occurrence and timing of bleeding and the duration of hospital stay.

For qualitative variables, analytical tools (frequency tables) and graphical tools (pie charts and bar charts) were used. For quantitative variables we used analytical tools such as location statistics (means and medians), dispersion (standard deviations, percentiles and ranges) and shape statistics (symmetry and kurtosis coefficient), as well as graphical tools (histograms and box plots).

The relationship of postoperative bleeding with each of the baseline variables, concomitant diseases and surgical characteristics was analyzed.

First, statistical tests were applied to see the relationship of each variable with surgical bleeding, and then an estimation of the risk of bleeding was carried out for each of the characteristics considered. Finally, logistic regression models were constructed to adjust the probability of bleeding according to each of the factors considered in the study.

The relationship of hospitalization time with each of the baseline variables, concomitant diseases, surgical characteristics and the presence of bleeding after surgery was analyzed.

Firstly, statistical tests were applied to see the relationship of each variable with the length of hospitalization. In this group of patients, the need for long hospitalisations is very low, so it was decided to recode the days of hospitalization as a categorical variable (one day vs. more than one day).

For all statistical analyses, the R software version 4.4.1 has been used. In all cases, bilateral tests have been applied using a significance level of 5%, obtaining exact p-values whenever possible.

3. Results

A total of 143 surgical procedures meeting the inclusion criteria were performed. Of these, 127 were carried out in oncologic patients (122 with squamous cell carcinoma and 5 with verrucous carcinoma) while the remaining 16 cases corresponded to other indications, such as unilateral vocal cord paralysis. The cohort was predominantly male (92%, n = 131), with a mean age of 65 years. Regarding exposure to toxic habits, 108 patients (75.5%) reported at least one: 84 (58.7%) were active smokers, and 71 (49.7%) consumed alcohol. Notably, 47 patients (32.9%) presented with both risk factors (Table 1).

Table 1. Demographics of the sample (SD: standard deviation; Min: minimum; Max: maximum; VCP: vocal cord paralysis; SCC: squamous cell carcinoma; VeC: verrucous carcinoma).

	Total
Total	143 (100%)
Sex	
Men	131 (91.6%)
Women	12 (8.4%)
Age	
Mean (SD)	65.1 (12.5)
Median (Min.–Max.)	66 (31–94)
<60 years	37 (25.9%)
60–69 years	50 (35.0%)
≥70 years	56 (39.2%)
Disease	
VCP	16 (11.2%)
SCC	122 (85.3%)
VeC	5 (3.5%)
Toxic habits	
No	35 (24.5%)
Yes	108 (75.5%)
Tobacco	84 (58.7%)
Alcohol	71 (49.7%)

Concerning comorbidities, 19.6% of patients (n = 28) had no associated medical conditions at the time of surgery. However, 80.4% (n = 115) presented with at least one concomitant disease. The most common subgroup consisted of patients with two comorbidities, accounting for 25.9% of the total. The most prevalent comorbidity was arterial hypertension, affecting 48% of patients, followed by dyslipidemia (39%), diabetes mellitus (17%), ischemic heart disease (15%), chronic obstructive pulmonary disease (12%), hypothyroidism (10%), anxiety-depressive syndrome (10%), other malignancies (8%), chronic venous insufficiency (6%), obesity (5%), bronchitis (5%), previous cerebrovascular events (5%), obstructive sleep apnea (5%), and peripheral arterial disease (1%) (Figure 1).

Regarding the type of surgical procedure performed, the majority of patients underwent a transmuscular cordectomy (Type III), accounting for 53.1% of cases. This was followed by extended cordectomy (Type V) in 44.1% of patients. A small subset underwent a complete cordectomy (Type IV), representing only 2.8% of the total (Figure 2).

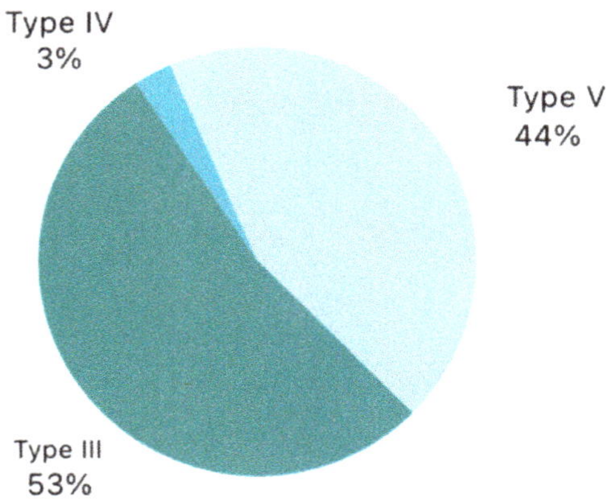

Figure 2. Types of cordectomies performed.

Additionally, seven patients (4.9%) were under anticoagulant therapy on the day of surgery, none of whom experienced postoperative bleeding.

A total of five postoperative bleeding events were recorded, corresponding to an estimated bleeding risk of 3.5% (95% CI: 1.5–7.9%) for this type of procedure performed with microelectrodes. The mean time to bleeding onset was 120 min after the end of surgery. The earliest case occurred immediately after extubation, while the latest occurred at 210 min postoperatively. No bleeding events were observed between 210 min and the seventh postoperative day, nor was any bleeding detected after the seventh postoperative day. Postoperative bleeding occurred in 8% of women and 3% of men. Four bleeding events were recorded in the oncologic group and one in the non-oncologic group. Approximately 5% of patients were under anticoagulant therapy; however, none of these patients experienced bleeding. Arterial hypertension was present in 49% of the total cohort, and 40% of the patients with bleeding had this condition. No statistically significant differences were found in postoperative bleeding by sex ($p = 0.359$), with an estimated risk of 3.1% in men (95% CI: 1.2–7.6%) and 8.3% in women (95% CI: 1.5–35.0%). Likewise, no significant difference was observed in median age between patients without bleeding (66 years) and those with bleeding (61 years) (p-value = 0.377). There was also no significant association between bleeding risk and underlying pathology (p-value = 0.554), with an estimated bleeding risk of 6.3% in patients with bilateral vocal cord paralysis and 3.3% in those with squamous cell carcinoma. No significant differences were observed based on smoking status (p-value = 0.649), with an estimated bleeding risk of 4.8% in smokers and 1.7% in non-smokers. Similarly, no significant differences were found with respect to alcohol consumption (p-value = 0.681), with an estimated bleeding risk of 4.2% in alcohol users and 2.8% in non-users. A statistically significant difference was observed in bleeding risk according to the type of cordectomy performed (p-value = 0.021), with no bleeding reported in patients who underwent a transmuscular cordectomy (Type III) and a 7.5% risk observed in those who underwent total or extended cordectomy (Type V). Patients undergoing Type IV–V cordectomies had an odds ratio of 13.464 for postoperative bleeding compared to those who underwent Type III procedures, a statistically significant result (p-value = 0.017). No other factors showed a statistically significant association in the univariate models, although bronchitis and sex demonstrated the highest levels of association among the remaining variables. These differences are illustrated in Figure 3.

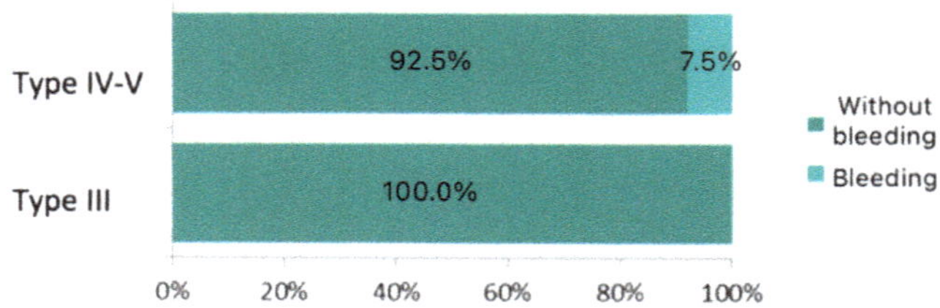

Figure 3. Percentage of bleeding by type of cordectomy.

Finally, the estimated bleeding risk was 0.0% in patients receiving anticoagulant therapy, compared to 3.7% in those not on such medication.

A multivariate model was constructed including those variables that showed a p-value < 0.25 in the univariate analysis. Table 2 summarizes the variables included in the univariate and multivariate analyses, indicating the level of statistical significance achieved with a 95% confidence interval.

Table 2. Summary of variables included in univariate and multivariate predictive model with an 95% confidence interval (CI) (SCC-VeC: squamous cell carcinoma–verrucous carcinoma; VCP: vocal cord paralysis).

Variable	Bleeding	No Bleeding	Univariate Model *p*-Value	Multivariate Model *p*-Value
Total-143 (100%)	5 (3.5%)	138 (96.5%)		
Type of cordectomy			0.017	0.005
Type III—transmuscular	0	76(100%)		
Type IV/V–total/extended	5 (7.5%)	62 (92.5%)		
Anticoagulant therapy			0.773	
No	5 (3.7%)	131 (96.3%)		
Yes	0 (0.0%)	7 (100%)		
Disease			0.357	
SCC-VeC VCP	123 (96.85%) 1 (6.3%)	4 (3.15%) 15 (93.8%)		
Sex			0.234	0.056
Men Women	4 (3.1%) 1 (8.3%)	127 (96.9%) 11 (91.7%)		
Age			0.571	
<60 years 60–69 years >70 years	1 (2.7%) 4 (8.0%) 0 (0.0%)	36 (97.3%) 46 (92.0%) 56 (100.0%)		
Smokers			0.391	
Yes No	4 (4.8%) 1 (1.7%)	80 (93.6%) 58 (98.3%)		
Alcoholism			0.663	
Yes No	2 (2.8%) 3 (4.2%)	68 (95.8%) 70 (97.2%)		
Chronic bronchitis			0.127	0.136
Yes No	1 (12.5%) 4 (30.0%)	7 (87.5%) 131 (97.0%)		

In the final model, the type of cordectomy emerged as the only statistically significant prognostic factor. However, factors such as gender (p = 0.056) and chronic bronchitis (p = 0.136) have also been included due to their proximity to statistical significance in the multivariate model, which increases its discriminatory power compared to the univariate model. All of this is reflected in Figure 4, which shows the ROC curve associated with the final multivariate predictive model, which demonstrates high discriminatory power, with an area under the curve (AUC) of 0.839—higher than that of the univariate model (AUC = 0.775).

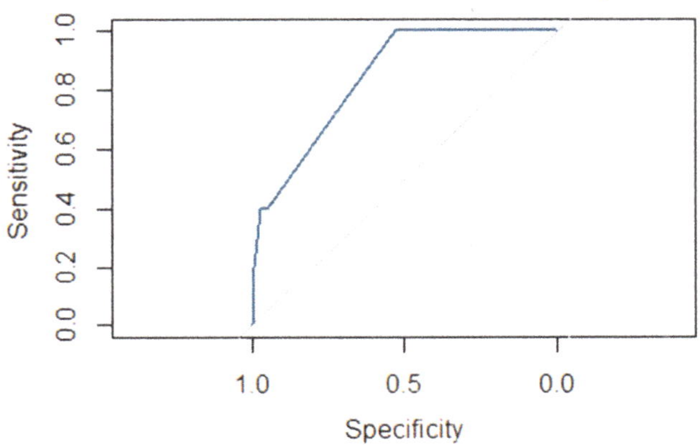

Figure 4. Predictive model for postoperative bleeding. The ROC curve associated with the final multivariate predictive model, which demonstrates high discriminatory power, with an area under the curve (AUC) of 0.839.

The mean hospital stay was 1.29 days, ranging from 1 to 7 days. Figure 5 illustrates the distribution of hospital stay duration in this patient cohort, showing that nearly all patients (87.4%) required only a single day of hospitalization.

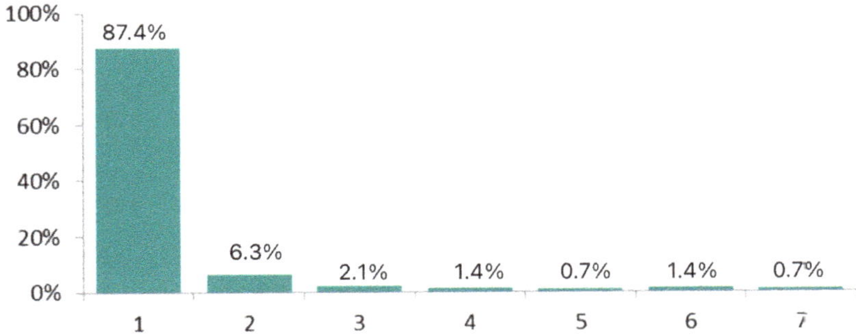

Figure 5. Days of hospitalization after surgery.

Although no statistically significant differences were observed, a trend was noted suggesting a relationship between smoking status and length of hospital stay (p-value = 0.105), with smokers exhibiting a longer hospitalization period compared to non-smokers.

Statistically significant differences were found in the number of hospitalization days based on the presence or absence of anxiety-depressive syndrome (p-value = 0.032).

Patients with ischemic heart disease also showed a tendency toward longer hospital stays, although this was not statistically significant (p-value = 0.119).

The type of cordectomy performed approached statistical significance in relation to hospitalization duration (p-value = 0.137), with longer stays observed in patients who underwent total or extended cordectomy.

Finally, a highly significant difference was observed in hospitalization time between patients who experienced surgical bleeding and those who did not (p-value < 0.001).

When constructing the multivariable predictive model, postoperative bleeding was identified as a significant predictor of hospital stay longer than one day (p-value < 0.001).

For the construction of this final penalized multivariate logistic regression model, factors with a significance level lower than 0.25 in the univariate model were included (smoking p = 0.083; ischaemic heart disease p = 0.144; anxiety–depression syndrome p = 0.088 and type of pathology p = 0.112) were included in the model, given that the small number of events observed makes it difficult to adjust models with many independent variables. Smoking status and the presence of certain comorbidities approached statistical significance and may reach significance with an expanded sample size. Figure 6 shows the ROC curve associated with the full multivariate predictive model including these variables, demonstrating good discriminative ability with an area under the curve (AUC) of 0.837. This performance surpasses that of the model including only postoperative bleeding, which had an AUC of 0.639. The improvement of the full model over the bleeding-only model was statistically significant (p-value < 0.001).

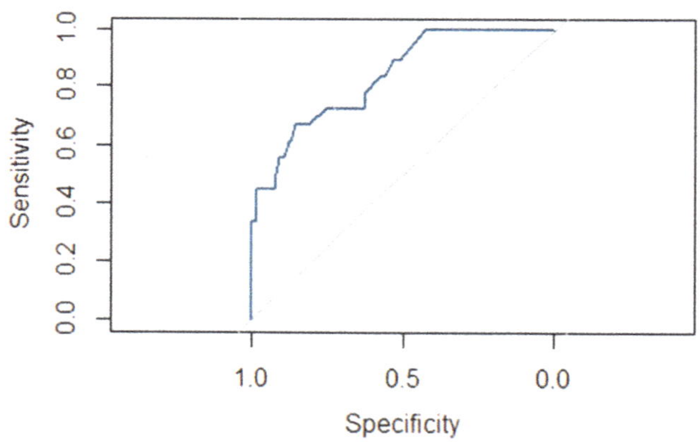

Figure 6. Predictive model for hospital stay. The ROC curve associated with the full multivariate predictive model including these variables, demonstrating good discriminative ability with an area under the curve (AUC) of 0.837.

Lastly, the costs incurred by the patients included in this study for the National Health System have been analyzed.

The total average cost per patient for outpatient cordectomy using TOMES was between EUR 963.82 and EUR 997.05, while procedures requiring hospitalization ranged from EUR 3523.15 to EUR 4651.67 (taking into account not only the surgery but also the stay in the post-anesthesia recovery unit, administrative costs, staff and materials). This represents an additional cost of between EUR 2559.33 and EUR 3688.85 when this surgery is performed on an inpatient basis, making inpatient surgery approximately 3.6 to 4.7 times more expensive than outpatient treatment. Assuming that hospitalization costs are the main factor explaining this difference, the excess cost corresponds to an estimated 2.3 to 4.1 days of post-surgical hospitalization (based on an average daily cost of between EUR

900 and EUR 1100). These results suggest that, although the surgical component itself is comparable, hospitalization significantly increases the total cost.

4. Discussion

The decision to perform a surgical procedure on an outpatient basis is inherently complex. It must take into account variables related to the underlying pathology, the surgical technique itself, the characteristics of the hospital, and, crucially, individual patient factors, both medical and social. These considerations guide the choice of the most appropriate and safest option for each patient, aiming to maximize well-being and potentially improve quality of life.

Before initiating outpatient surgical planning, it is essential to review the ambulatory surgery eligibility criteria specific to the institution. These typically include optimal control of chronic diseases, availability of adequate postoperative surveillance during the first 24 h, access to private transportation to the nearest hospital equipped to manage postoperative complications, and the patient's proximity to that facility. Once these criteria are met, case-by-case evaluation allows us to offer safe outpatient surgery on an individual and personalized basis for each patient.

Over 80% of patients presented with at least one comorbidity, with arterial hypertension being the most common, present in nearly half of the cohort. This is a relevant finding considering the historical association between hypertension and increased risk of systemic bleeding [13]. However, in our analysis, the presence of hypertension did not correlate with a higher postoperative bleeding risk when cordectomies were performed using the TOMES technique. Combined with the low incidence of bleeding within the first 7 postoperative days, these results support the inclusion of well-controlled hypertensive patients in outpatient surgery protocols.

A similar trend was observed in anticoagulated patients. Although anticoagulant therapy, as well as coagulopathies or other haemostatic disorders, is classically associated with increased bleeding risk [14], our findings suggest that, with appropriate perioperative management, these patients did not experience a significantly higher incidence of bleeding when treated with the TOMES approach.

No bleeding events were observed beyond 210 min postoperatively. This suggests that there is no need to extend the usual postoperative recovery room monitoring time, which typically ranges from 6 to 8 h in most ambulatory surgical procedures. Furthermore, to ensure patient safety, no bleeding events were recorded between 210 min postoperatively and the 7th postoperative day in our sample. In other words, no haemorrhagic complications occurred at home after hospital discharge.

No statistically significant differences were observed in bleeding risk based on the underlying pathology (glottic carcinoma vs. vocal cord paralysis). Although bilateral vocal fold paralysis is not typically considered a risk factor for increased bleeding, in this study, a higher proportion of bleeding events was observed in these cases. This finding may be influenced by the relatively small number of patients with this pathology included in the cohort compared to those with tumoral lesions.

This finding warrants further investigation in future studies, as tumoral pathologies are generally associated with a higher bleeding tendency due to their rich vascularization, which often includes aberrant and fragile vessels [15].

While no significant differences were observed in bleeding risk by sex, smoking, chronic bronchitis, obesity, diabetes, dyslipidemia, etc., a statistically significant association was found between the type of cordectomy and postoperative bleeding. Specifically, extended cordectomies (Types IV and V), which involve resection beyond a single vocal fold [8,9], were associated with a 7.5% higher risk of bleeding. This finding is consistent with the expected increase in vascular injury in more extensive resections, especially when optimal haemostasis is not achieved. It is also possible that this association is indirectly related to tumour size, as larger tumours typically require more extensive surgical resections, which, as observed in this study, are associated with an increased risk of postoperative bleeding.

Other previously discussed variables, such as sex, chronic bronchitis, and smoking status, did not reach statistical significance; however, a trend toward significance was observed in relation to an increased risk of postoperative bleeding. These factors may potentially influence bleeding outcomes but the limited number of bleeding events and the overall low incidence of this complication in TOMES cordectomies may have reduced the power to detect significant differences.

For these reasons, developing and applying an individualized risk prediction model for postoperative bleeding is a valuable next step. Expanding the sample size in future studies will allow for a more refined analysis of variables that, while not statistically significant in the current cohort, have shown clinically relevant trends.

Although transoral laser cordectomies have been performed on an outpatient basis in some centres for years [16], cordectomies performed using transoral robotic surgery (TORS) have only recently been introduced, and indications for this surgical approach are steadily increasing. Furthermore, an expanding number of centres are incorporating this technique into their clinical practice [17].

Because of these reasons, this predictive risk model would not only be applicable when using microelectrodes as the surgical instrument but could also be extrapolated to optimize patient selection for transoral laser [16] or TORS cordectomies [17]. In doing so, it would contribute to optimizing outpatient surgical pathways and enhancing safety in procedures involving the upper airway.

Furthermore, we analyzed hospital length of stay in this cohort, aiming to identify which factors may contribute to prolonged hospitalization, particularly relevant given the known increase in hospitalization and elevated complications associated with extended inpatient stays. Postoperative bleeding was significantly associated with a longer hospital stay, as additional days of monitoring are required to ensure adequate haemostasis and optimal recovery. However, bleeding was not the only factor contributing to prolonged hospitalization. Other relevant risk factors were identified that should also be considered in the preoperative assessment. As discussed earlier, more extensive surgeries, which are often required for larger tumours, are associated with a higher risk of bleeding and, indirectly, with longer hospital stays due to the need for extended surveillance. Although not reaching statistical significance, a clear trend toward longer hospital stays was observed in smokers, patients with ischemic heart disease, and those with anxiety-depressive disorders. In the multivariable logistic regression model, the risk of prolonged hospitalization was notably higher in patients presenting with one or more of these four risk factors. These patient characteristics should therefore be incorporated into a predictive model for hospital length of stay.

On the other hand, transoral laser cordectomies have been associated with lower treatment costs for T1–T2 glottic tumours compared to open cordectomy or radiotherapy [5]. In addition, it is important to highlight the economic savings achieved by performing this surgery using transoral microelectrode surgery (TOMES) instead of laser, while still offering comparable clinical outcomes [6]. Furthermore, this study has shown how outpatient care significantly reduces the cost per patient, resulting in savings equivalent to the cost of a hospital stay of between 2 and 4 days per patient. This represents a significant reduction in healthcare expenses, which in turn has a positive impact on the National Health System.

In summary, both individual predictive models, one for bleeding risk and another hospital stay duration, are promising tools that must be used with caution. Their predictive power should be validated and refined over time as the dataset grows and more events are recorded. With this approach, patients can be appropriately selected for outpatient TOMES cordectomies based on their individual profiles, contributing to reduced surgical wait times, fewer hospital admissions, and overall lower healthcare costs. Additionally, minimizing hospital stay may help reduce the incidence of inpatient complications and promote a more comfortable surgical experience for patients, ultimately improving their quality of life.

5. Conclusions

Cordectomies performed via transoral microelectrode surgery (TOMES) are common procedures routinely carried out in hospital settings. Type III, IV, and V cordectomies performed using this technique have demonstrated a low rate of immediate postoperative bleeding complications. In this series, the latest bleeding event occurred 3.5 h after surgery, suggesting that selected cases can be safely managed in an outpatient setting with an appropriately postoperative monitoring. Moreover, extended cordectomies have been associated with a higher risk of bleeding.

When considering this approach, it is essential to make individualized decisions using a personalized predictive model that incorporates patient-specific risk factors, comorbidities, and the planned type of cordectomy. This strategy has the potential to improve patient quality of life and reduce healthcare costs.

Author Contributions: Conceptualization, E.Z.; methodology, E.F.-V., J.R.A.-G. and E.Z.; investigation, C.R.-P., E.F.-V., J.R.A.-G. and E.Z.; resources, C.R.-P.; data curation, C.R.-P. and E.F.-V.; writing—original draft preparation, C.R.-P. and N.O.; writing—review and editing, N.O., E.F.-V., J.R.A.-G. and E.Z.; supervision, J.R.A.-G.; project administration, N.O. All authors have read and agreed to the published version of the manuscript.

Funding: This research received no external funding.

Institutional Review Board Statement: The study was conducted according to the guidelines of the Declaration of Helsinki and approved by the Ethics Committee of the General University Hospital of Valencia (protocol 38/2023, approved on 26 May 2023). The Ethics Committee has approved the collection of data for the whole of 2023.

Informed Consent Statement: Patient consent was waived due to retrospective design and anonymity guarantee. The study involved only anonymized data from past procedures, with no additional interventions or risks to patients.

Data Availability Statement: Data is contained within the article.

Conflicts of Interest: The authors declare no conflicts of interest.

ferences

SEER. Cancer of the Larynx—Cancer Stat Facts. Available online: https://seer.cancer.gov/statfacts/html/laryn.html (accessed on 1 September 2024).

Feng, Y.; Wang, B.; Wen, S. Laser surgery versus radiotherapy for T1–T2N0 glottic cancer: A meta-analysis. *ORL J. Otorhino-Laryngol. Relat. Spec.* **2011**, *73*, 336–342. [CrossRef] [PubMed]

3. Vaculik, M.F.; MacKay, C.A.; Taylor, S.M.; Trites, J.R.B.; Hart, R.D.; Rigby, M.H. Systematic review and meta-analysis of T1 glc cancer outcomes comparing CO_2 transoral laser microsurgery and radiotherapy. *J. Otolaryngol.-Head Neck Surg.* **2019**, *48* [CrossRef] [PubMed]
4. Baird, B.J.; Sung, C.K.; Beadle, B.M.; Divi, V. Treatment of early-stage laryngeal cancer: A comparison of treatment options. C *Oncol.* **2018**, *87*, 8–16. [CrossRef] [PubMed]
5. Diaz-De-Cerio, P.; Preciado, J.; Santaolalla, F.; Sanchez-Del-Rey, A. Cost-minimisation and cost-effectiveness analysis compar transoral CO_2 laser cordectomy, laryngofissure cordectomy and radiotherapy for the treatment of T1–2, N0, M0 glottic carcino *Eur. Arch. Oto-Rhino-Laryngol.* **2013**, *270*, 1181–1188. [CrossRef] [PubMed]
6. Basterra, J.; Zapater, E.; Moreno, R.; Hernández, R. Electrosurgical endoscopic cordectomy with microdissection electrodes comparative study with CO_2 laser. *J. Laryngol. Otol.* **2006**, *120*, 661–664. [CrossRef] [PubMed]
7. Weingarten, T.N.; Bojanić, K.; Scavonetto, F.; Sprung, J. Management of delayed hemorrhage after partial vocal cord cordecto *J. Clin. Anesth.* **2013**, *25*, 666–668. [CrossRef] [PubMed]
8. Remacle, M.; Eckel, H.E.; Antonelli, A.; Brasnu, D.; Chevalier, D.; Friedrich, G.; Olofsson, J.; Rudert, H.H.; Thumfart, W.; Vincentiis, M.; et al. Endoscopic cordectomy: A proposal for a classification by the working committee, European Laryngolog Society. *Eur. Arch. Oto-Rhino-Laryngol.* **2000**, *257*, 227–231. [CrossRef] [PubMed]
9. Remacle, M.; Van Haverbeke, C.; Eckel, H.; Bradley, P.; Chevalier, D.; Djukic, V.; de Vicentiis, M.; Friedrich, G.; Olofsson, J.; Per G.; et al. Proposal for revision of the European Laryngological Society classification of endoscopic cordectomies. *Eur. A Oto-Rhino-Laryngol.* **2007**, *264*, 499–504. [CrossRef] [PubMed]
10. Poves-Álvarez, R.; Gómez-Sánchez, E.; Martínez-Rafael, B.; Bartolomé, C.; Alvarez-Fuente, E.; Muñoz-Moreno, M.F.; Eiros, J Tamayo, E.; Gómez-Pesquera, E. Parental satisfaction with autonomous pediatric ambulatory surgery units. *Qual. Manag. He Care* **2021**, *30*, 145–152. [CrossRef] [PubMed]
11. Nordin, A.B.; Shah, S.R.; Kenney, B.D. Ambulatory pediatric surgery. *Semin. Pediatr. Surg.* **2018**, *27*, 75–78. [CrossRef] [PubM
12. Dor, A.; Luo, Q.; Gerstein, M.T.; Malveaux, F.; Mitchell, H.; Markus, A.R. Cost-effectiveness of an Evidence-Based Childhc Asthma Intervention in Real-World Primary Care Settings. *J. Ambul. Care Manag.* **2018**, *41*, 213–224. [CrossRef] [PubMed]
13. Vogel, B.; Mehran, R. Arterial hypertension: A neglected risk for bleeding. *Catheter. Cardiovasc. Interv.* **2016**, *88*, 191– [CrossRef] [PubMed]
14. Proietti, M.; Romiti, G.F.; Romanazzi, I.; Farcomeni, A.; Staerk, L.; Nielsen, P.B.; Lip, G.Y. Restarting oral anticoagulant thera after major bleeding in atrial fibrillation: A systematic review and meta-analysis. *Int. J. Cardiol.* **2018**, *261*, 84–91. [CrossR [PubMed]
15. Olszewski, E. Blood Vascular System in Cancer of the Larynx. *Arch. Otolaryngol.* **1976**, *102*, 65–70. [CrossRef] [PubMed]
16. Altuna, X.; Zulueta, A.; Algaba, J. CO_2 laser cordectomy as a day-case procedure. *J. Laryngol. Otol.* **2005**, *119*, 770–773. [CrossR [PubMed]
17. Hans, S.; Baudouin, R.; Circiu, M.P.; Couineau, F.; Lisan, Q.; Crevier-Buchman, L.; Lechien, J.R. Laryngeal Cancer Surgery: Hist and Current Indications of Transoral Laser Microsurgery and Transoral Robotic Surgery. *J. Clin. Med.* **2022**, *11*, 5769. [CrossR [PubMed]

Journal of
Personalized Medicine

MDPI

ematic Review

elphi Consensus in Otolaryngology: A Systematic Review of eliability and Reporting Completeness

astasia Urbanelli [1,†], Giorgia Pugliese [2,†], Elisa Bolis [2], Matilde Coccapani [2], Martina Gemma Corti [2], bara D'Angelo [2], Anna Lancieri [2], Laura Maggi [2], Antonino Maniaci [3,4], Jerome R. Lechien [4]
Alberto Maria Saibene [2,4,*]

1 Division of Otorhinolaryngology, Department of Surgical Sciences, Università degli Studi di Torino, 10124 Turin, Italy; anastasia.urbanelli@unito.it
2 Otolaryngology Unit, Santi Paolo E Carlo Hospital, Department of Health Sciences, Università Degli Studi Di Milano, 20142 Milan, Italy; elisa.bolis@unimi.it (E.B.)
3 Faculty of Medicine and Surgery, University of Enna "Kore", 94100 Enna, Italy
4 Department of Surgery, UMONS Research Institute for Health Sciences and Technology, University of Mons (UMons), 7000 Mons, Belgium; jerome.lechien@umons.ac.be
* Correspondence: alberto.saibene@unimi.it; Tel.: +39-02-8184-4249
† These authors contributed equally to this work.

Abstract: Background: The Delphi method is increasingly used in otolaryngology to develop consensus in subjects lacking robust evidence. In these contexts, consensus documents play a dual role: they provide structured expert guidance while determining shared principles adaptable to the individual patient. Nevertheless, the methodological rigor and reporting consistency of Delphi studies remain variable, raising concerns about transparency, reproducibility, and potential bias. **Methods:** A systematic review was conducted according to PRISMA guidelines. MEDLINE, Embase, and Web of Science were searched for Delphi-based consensus studies in otolaryngology. Fully published studies in English, Italian, German, French, or Spanish were included. Each article was assessed using established methodological frameworks for consensus development, bias domains described in the methodological literature, and the DELPHISTAR reporting checklist. Reliability and completeness scores were calculated to enable comparisons. **Results:** Out of 3168 unique records, 86 studies were included. Most defined their purpose and consensus criteria, but transparency regarding panel selection, anonymity, feedback, and criteria for stopping the consensus process was often missing. Based on methodological bias domains, only 9 studies (10.5%) reached a "good" reliability score, while the majority were rated as "fair." According to DELPHISTAR, just 3 studies (3.5%) showed good levels of completeness. Reporting completeness and risk of bias proved heterogeneous across subspecialties. **Conclusions:** Delphi-based studies are increasingly shaping clinical practice in otolaryngology, but persistent methodological and reporting limitations undermine their reliability. Wider adoption of standardized frameworks is essential to improve transparency, reproducibility, and clinical impact, ensuring that consensus statements support both evidence-informed practice and personalized patient care.

Keywords: guidelines; consensus; Delphi; methodology; bias; quality evaluation; otolaryngology

1. Introduction

The "Delphi method" (DeMet) is a structured, group-based process used to achieve consensus among a panel of experts through multiple rounds of questionnaires. After each round, participants receive anonymous feedback summarizing the group's responses, allowing them to revise their views in subsequent rounds. This iterative process continues until a stable consensus is reached [1].

Throughout the years, the adoption of this technique has become increasingly common for forecasting, decision-making, and developing guidelines, especially in situations where evidence is limited or uncertain [2]. The DeMet is mostly used in studies involving medicine, technology, natural science, and behavioral social sciences [3].

In medicine, Delphi-based consensus statements play a particularly crucial role, as they often represent the only structured framework available to guide clinical decisions in fields where robust evidence is scarce. In these contexts, consensus is not only a pragmatic substitute for guidelines but also a foundation for delivering personalized care: it allows clinicians to rely on expert-derived principles while tailoring therapeutic strategies to the specific needs of individual patients. This dual role makes consensus documents a cornerstone of modern personalized medicine, bridging the gap between limited evidence and the demand for individualized, evidence-informed treatments.

Given the widespread interest in the DeMet in the research field, especially in topics lacking strong evidence, several reporting guidelines have been introduced to improve methodological transparency and consistency. Notable among these is the CREDES (Guidance on Conducting and REporting DElphi Studies) [4], which provides practical recommendations for both the design and reporting of Delphi studies to ensure methodological transparency and reproducibility, and ACCORD (ACcurate COnsensus Reporting Document), which focuses on standardizing how consensus-based research is documented and interpreted [5]. However, both protocols have shown significant limitations, particularly in addressing the diversity of Delphi applications and methodological variants. To overcome these gaps, the DELPHI-STAR (Studies in The Areas of Reporting) guidelines [6] were developed, offering the most comprehensive and interdisciplinary standard currently available for reporting Delphi studies. As a result, studies interpreting the risk of bias for DeMet studies have emerged [7], allowing for a more reproducible appropriateness and reliability evaluation.

The growing adoption of the DeMet across various disciplines (including otolaryngology) highlights the need for a rigorous and standardized methodological framework: this need is also acknowledged by the AAO-HNSF (American Academy of Otolaryngology–Head and Neck Surgery Foundation) [2].

In this context, the present study carried out a systematic review of Delphi-based publications in otolaryngology to evaluate how rigorously the DeMet has been applied in the field and to identify examples of best practices as well as recurring methodological limitations. The primary aim of this systematic review is to promote more rigorous methodological standards that enhance the overall impact, clinical relevance, and scientific validity of Delphi research in this field.

2. Materials and Methods

This review can be found in The Open Science Framework with DOI (https://doi.org/10.17605/OSF.IO/8CXS7). Following protocol registration in the Open Science Framework database [8], we conducted a systematic review between 17 September 2024, and 5 May 2025, in accordance with the PRISMA reporting guidelines [9]. The PRISMA checklist is provided in Supplementary Table S1. Systematic electronic searches were performed in English, Italian, German, French, and Spanish to identify any Delphi-method consensus published on topics of otolaryngological interest.

On 17 September 2024, we conducted a primary search on the MEDLINE, Embase, and Web of Science databases. The search terms used were as follows: delphi AND (otolaryngolog* OR otorhinolaryngolog* OR otolog* OR rhinolog* OR laryngolog* OR audiolog* OR phoniatric* OR nose* OR nasal* OR paranasal* OR sinus* OR mouth* OR pharyn* OR laryngopharyn* OR nasopharyn* OR oropharyn* OR rhinopharyn* OR hypopharyn* OR throat* OR larynx OR laryngeal OR "vocal cord*" OR "vocal fold*" OR ear OR ears OR neck* OR salivary OR adenoid* OR tonsil* OR tongue* OR speech OR hearing OR audition* OR deglutition* OR swallow* OR respiration* OR breathing OR gustation* OR taste OR smell* OR olfaction* OR sinusitis OR rhinosinusit* OR tonsilliti* OR otiti* OR rhinitis* OR ototoxic* OR sleep* OR apnea* OR OSA OR Epistaxis OR rhinorrhea OR rhinorrea OR deafness OR hypoacus* OR hoarse* OR dysphagia OR xerostomia* OR hyposalivation* OR hyposialia).

Additionally, we planned to manually examine the references for selected publications to identify any further relevant reports not retrieved by the initial database search.

Only fully published Delphi-method consensus were considered for inclusion.

Exclusion criteria were as follows:

- Non-human studies;
- Non-otolaryngology-related Delphi topic;
- Papers published in languages other than English, Italian, German, French, or Spanish;
- Conference abstracts;
- Protocol-only papers;
- Studies using mixed consensus techniques or using the DeMet for purposes other than obtaining a clinical consensus (e.g., using Delphi for prioritizing items in a list);
- Studies published before the Rosenfeld development manual appeared in the literature [2];
- Studies lacking an otolaryngologist in the development group or with less than 50% otolaryngologists among panelists.

Abstract and full-text reviews were conducted in duplicate by different authors. During the abstract review stage, all studies deemed eligible by at least one reviewer were included. Disagreements during the full-text review stage were resolved through consensus among the reviewers.

The PICOTS framework did not apply to this study, as its research methodology was not focused on patient populations.

Data extraction and study rating were performed in duplicate by two authors, with discrepancies resolved through consensus.

Based on the frameworks developed by Rosenfeld et al. [2], Nasa et al. [7], and the DELPHISTAR initiative [6], each study was evaluated to assess its alignment with established standards for consensus-building research, to obtain a synthesized overview of the quality of the articles examined.

For each article included, the following outcomes were recorded:

- The related otolaryngology subspecialty (if applicable);
- Key elements such as planning, development, and structure according to the Rosenfeld development manual (defining scope, development group, appropriate literature review, modified DeMet implementation, panel inclusion criteria, number of drafting and revision rounds, number of statements, and final results) for a total of 7 items;
- Potential bias elements according to Nasa et al. [7]. (identification of problem area, selection of panel members, anonymity of panelists, controlled feedback, iterative rounds, consensus criteria analysis of consensus, closing criteria, i.e., the criteria which define when the consensus process should be stopped without further rounds, stability) for a total of 9 items;

- Reporting completeness according to the Delphistar protocol (38 items).

The quality assessment, which is usually a key component of a systematic review, was essentially the core component of the data extraction process and represented the primary objective of the article itself, which was specifically designed to evaluate both the reliability and completeness of reporting. Therefore, the quality appraisal is inherently embedded within those processes.

Due to the predominantly qualitative nature of the collected data, no initial or subsequent meta-analysis was planned or conducted.

In order to allow easier comparisons of the results, after evaluating each article for reliability and potential bias according to the Nasa et al. [7]. work and reporting completeness according to the Delphistar protocol, we devised and assigned a specific score.

Regarding the Nasa et al. [7]. protocol, we reported for each article a reliability score given as the percentage of the items not at risk of bias out of the nine proposed. In case an item could not be applied to a specific article (as it was often the case for the "stability" item), such an item was ignored for the overall score.

Based on the score achieved, the articles have been subsequently classified for reliability and potential bias as follows: poor: less than 35% of items not at risk of bias; fair: between 35−70% of items not at risk of bias; good: >70% of items not at risk of bias.

Following an analogous method, we also scored each article for the completeness achieved according to the Delphistar protocol and expressed it as a percentage based on the 38 proposed items. In case an item could not be applied to a particular article, such as "Information about the sources of funding" and "Justification of the Delphi variation and modifications", those items were excluded.

Based on the score achieved, the articles' completeness was subsequently classified as follows: very poor: less than 25% of items reported; poor: 25−50% of items reported; fair: 50−75% of items reported; good >70% of items reported.

3. Results

Among the 3,168 unique research items initially identified, 271 published reports were selected for full-text evaluation. No further report was identified for full-text evaluation after reference checking. Ultimately, a total of 86 articles were retained for analysis (see Figure 1). The list of DeMet consensus included in this systematic review is provided in Supplementary Material Table S2.

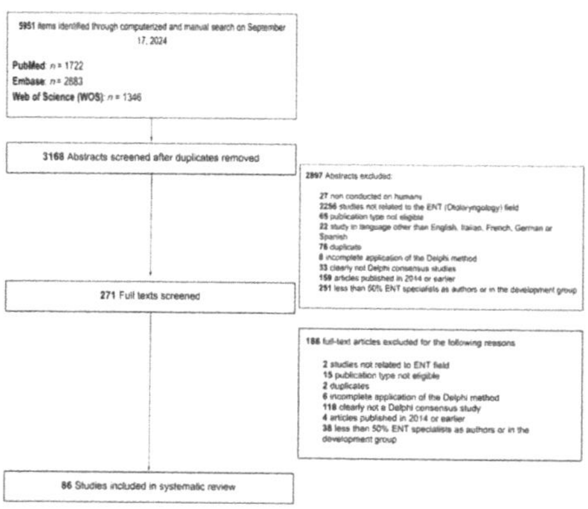

Figure 1. Delphi-style flowchart depicting the article selection process.

The literature was categorized according to the otolaryngology field covered: skull base, otology, laryngology, neuromonitoring, nose and paranasal sinuses, head and neck oncology, sleep and apnea, pediatric otolaryngology, thyroid, and "other". Items retrieved for each otolaryngology topic are detailed in Table 1.

Table 1. Topic-based categorization of the articles included in the systematic review.

Topic	No. of DeMet Consensuses Identified
Skull base	4
Ear	6
Laryngology	13
Neuromonitoring	2
Nose and paranasal sinuses	15
Head and neck oncology	13
Sleep/apnea	2
Pediatric otolaryngology	17
Thyroid	9
Other	5

The table reports the number of articles included in this systematic review according to the main topic. The section "other" includes topics addressed by a single article unclassifiable in the other sections.

3.1. *Application of Rosenfeld's Methodology*

All the 86 analyzed studies predetermined the purpose of the consensus according to Rosenfeld's development manual; 65 performed and documented a literature review before the consensus, while 2 explicitly did not, and 19 did not declare it. Regarding the implementation method, 33 studies applied the classic modified method, 22 the Rosenfeld method, 15 the Nominal Group Technique (NGT), and 16 other methodologies.

The development group was explicitly described in 66 out of 86 articles: of these, 43 included an exclusively otolaryngological development group, and in 22, it was a mixed (otolaryngological and non-otolaryngological) group. A single included DeMet consensus had a completely non-otolaryngological development group. Regarding the panel, 70 articles specified the number of panelists, with a mean value of 28.7 members (median 25, interquartile range 17.75, min 7, max 125). A total of 53 articles reported a multispecialty panel group; in 29, it was an exclusively otolaryngological panel, while 4 articles did not define the clinical specialty of panel members.

84 out of 86 articles defined the number of drafting and revision rounds, with a mean value of 2.6 (median 2.5, IQR 1, min 1, max 5). 81 articles reported the number of initial and final statements. Initial statements were 50.28 on average (median 25, IQR 32, range 4–413). Approved statements were 30.76 on average (median 21, interquartile range 23, range 4–133).

3.2. *Potential Bias Elements*

In the evaluation conducted following Nasa et al. [7]. appropriateness criteria, 83 out of 86 articles correctly identified the problem area. The selection of panel members' criteria was explicit in 47 out of 86 articles, whilst anonymity of the panelists was guaranteed only in 26 articles, with 21 articles being unclear. Controlled feedback was referred to in 6 articles, with 17 studies being unclear, whilst iterative rounds were recorded in 80 articles. Consensus criteria were established in 81 articles; analysis of consensus was described in

64. Closing criteria were established in only 16 articles, and stability in 11. Table 2 reports the reliability score of the included articles. Figure 2 provides a graphical synthesis of the same values.

Table 2. Article reliability.

Reliability Score According to Nasa et al. [7].								
1 Identification of problem area	2 Selection of panel members	3 Anonymity of panelists	4 Controlled feedback	5 Iterative rounds	6 Consensus criteria	7 Analysis of consensus	8 Closing criteria	9 Stability
1/9	1/9	1/9	1/9	1/9	1/9	1/9	1/9	1/9
Total = 9/9 *								
Reliability (% of total)				Poor: score < 35%				n = 12
				Fair: score 35–70%				n = 65
				Good: score > 70%				n = 9

The table reports the 9 items of the Nasa et al. [7]. evaluation for bias and the reliability score. * If an item could not be applied to a specific article, it was ignored for the overall score.

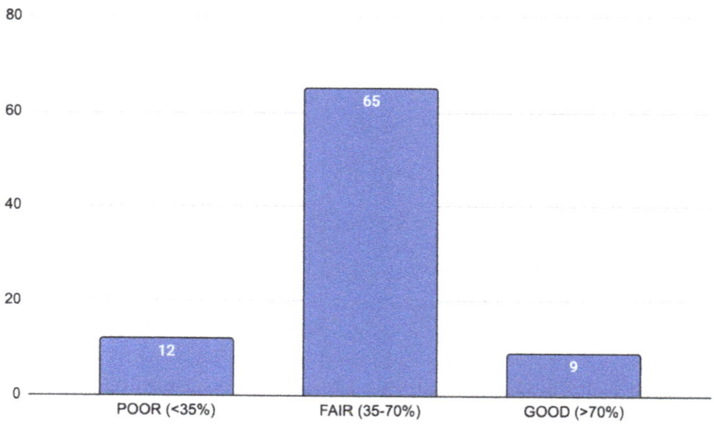

Figure 2. Reliability score of articles according to Nasa et al. [7]. Whenever an item could not be applied to a specific article, it was ignored for the overall score.

3.3. Application of the DELPHISTAR Reporting Framework

3.3.1. Title and Abstract

In 16 of the examined articles, the Delphi procedure was identified in the title, while 81 in the Delphi procedure appeared in the abstract. A total of 60 studies had a structured abstract, while 26 lacked such structuring.

3.3.2. Context

The context group was subdivided into "formal" and "content" related criteria. Considering the formal-related criteria, 30 articles provided information about the sources of funding; 40 articles provided details about the team of authors and researchers, specifying the discipline and the institution; information about method consulting was made explicit in 11 articles, while information about the project background was provided in a total of 63 papers. Lastly, the study protocol was explicit in a total of 19 articles.

Regarding the content-related criteria, the justification of the chosen method to execute the consensus was explicit in 18 articles, while the aim of the Delphi procedure was written down in all the scientific productions.

3.3.3. Method

The method criteria were divided into the following subgroups: body and integration of knowledge, Delphi variations, sample of experts, survey, Delphi rounds, feedback, and data analysis.

In the first subgroup, we checked if there was identification and elucidation of relevant expertise, spheres of experience, and perspectives, which were present in 58 papers; only 9 articles missed or deliberately not integrated handling of knowledge, expertise, and perspectives; lastly, in 17 studies, we found a proper definition of an expert.

Delphi variations subgroup: there was an identification of the type of Delphi procedure and potential modifications in 70 papers; in 10 studies, there was a justification of the Delphi variation and modifications, while in 5, it was not applicable, and in the remaining 71, this was not performed.

Regarding the sample of experts: in 64 articles, the selection criteria for the experts were presented; in 85, there was the identification of the experts, and in 5.9, there was information about recruiting and any subsequent recruitment of experts.

For the survey, the elucidation of the content development for the questionnaire was performed in 83 publications, while the description of the questions with their content and structure was performed in 84 articles.

Regarding the number of Delphi rounds: they went from a minimum of 1 to a maximum of 5, with a mean value of 2.6 (median 3, IQR 3 − 2). However, the number of Delphi rounds was not explicit in 2 papers. Information about the aims of the individual Delphi rounds was discussed in 35 of the studies, and the disclosure and justification of the criteria for discontinuation were conducted for 15 scientific productions.

In the feedback subgroup, we checked if there was any information about what data was reported back per round, and this was performed in 38 studies. 13 publications specified how the results of the previous Delphi round were fed back to the experts surveyed; it could be via frequencies, mean values, measures of dispersion, listing of comments, at the same time 3 papers specified whether feedback was differentiated by specific groups. Finally, 22 papers clarified how dissent and unclear results were handled.

Data analysis practices were one of the most concerning areas: only 2 studies outlined a detailed qualitative and quantitative strategy. However, a definition of consensus was provided much more frequently in 71 studies. Only three articles addressed weighting or subgroup analysis in their interpretation of the results.

3.3.4. Results

The results criteria were subdivided into the Delphi process and the results.

Taking into consideration the Delphi process criteria, the illustration of the Delphi process was provided by 23 publications, while 8 papers reported information about any special aspects during the Delphi process. The number of experts per round, both invited and participating, was indicated in 54 cases.

Finally, for the results, we can consult the presentation of the results for each Delphi round and the final results for the 39 papers.

3.3.5. Discussion

The discussion criteria are related to the quality of findings. Despite 66 studies highlighting the value of their findings, no one addressed the validity or potential transferability of their conclusions. Only 31 studies offered a critical reflection on the methodological limitations, and not a single publication attempted to assess inter-rater reliability or reproduce findings through split-panel comparisons. Table 3 reports analytic completeness data for all included articles. Figure 3 provides a graphical synthesis of the same values.

Table 3. Article completeness.

DELPHISTAR Completeness Score		
1 Title and abstract	Identification as a Delphi procedure in the title; Identification as a Delphi procedure in the abstract; Structured abstract	Tot: 3/38
2 Context	Formal: information about the sources of funding *; the team of authors and/or researchers; method consulting; the project background; the study protocol	Tot: 5/38
	Content: justification of the chosen method (Delphi procedure) to answer the research question; aim of the Delphi procedure (e.g., consensus, forecasting)	Tot: 2/38
3 Method	Body and integration of knowledge: Identification and elucidation of relevant expertise, spheres of experience, and perspectives; handling of knowledge, expertise and perspectives which are missing or have been deliberately not integrated; basic definition of expert	Tot: 3/38
	Delphi variations: Identification of the type of Delphi procedure and potential modifications; justification of the Delphi variation and modifications *, including during the Delphi process, if applicable *	Tot: 2/38
	Sample of experts: Selection criteria; Identification of the experts; Information about recruitment and any subsequent recruitment of experts	Tot: 3/38
	Survey: Elucidation of the content development for the questionnaire; Description of the questionnaire	Tot: 2/38
	Delphi rounds: Number of rounds; Information about the aims of the individual Delphi rounds; Disclosure and justification of the criterion for discontinuation	Tot: 3/38
	Feedback: Information about what data was reported back per round; Information on how the results of the previous round were fed back to the experts surveyed; Information on whether feedback was differentiated by specific groups; Information about how dissent and unclear results were handled	Tot: 4/38
	Data analysis: Disclosure of the quantitative and qualitative analytical strategy; Definition and measurement of consensus; Information on group-specific analysis or weighting of experts	Tot: 3/38
4 Results	Delphi process: Illustration of the Delphi process; Information about special aspects during the Delphi process; Number of experts per round (both invited and participating)	Tot: 3/38
	Results: Presentation of the results for each Delphi round and the final results	Tot: 1/38
5 Discussion	Quality of findings: Highlighting the findings from the Delphi study; Validity of the results; Reliability of the results; Reflection on potential limitations	Tot: 4/38
	Total = 38/38 *	

Table 3. *Cont.*

DELPHISTAR Completeness Score		
Completeness (% of total)	Very poor: score < 25%;	n = 1
	Poor: score 25–50%;	n = 38
	Fair: score 50–75%;	n = 44
	Good: score > 70%	n = 3

The table reports the 38 items of the DELPHISTAR protocol and the article completeness score. * If an item could not be applied to a specific article, it was ignored for the overall score.

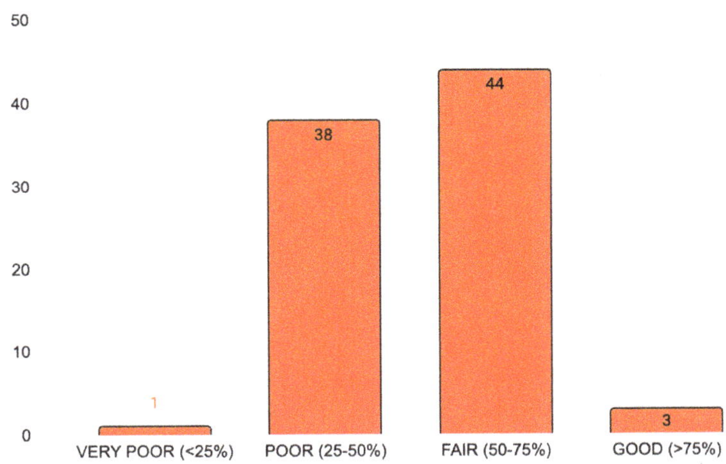

Figure 3. Article completeness score according to the DELPHISTAR protocol. X-axis: classification; Y-axis: total number of articles included.

3.4. Overall Evaluation

3.4.1. Reliability and Potential Bias According to Nasa et al. [7]

In terms of appropriateness and reliability, 12 articles were classified as "poor", having a reliability score < 35%; 65 articles were classified as "fair" (score equal to 35–70%), and finally, only 9 articles were classified as "good" (score > 70%).

3.4.2. Delphistar Reporting Completeness Score

In terms of reporting completeness, only 1 article was rated very poor (score < 25%); 38 articles were rated poor (score from 25 to 50%); 44 articles were rated fair (score 50–75%), and 3 articles were rated good, with a score > 70%.

4. Discussion

In recent decades, the DeMet has been widely applied across multiple disciplines, particularly in the medical and natural sciences, as well as in the behavioral and social sciences [6]. Owing to its strong ability to integrate expert opinion with available evidence, the DeMet is frequently adopted in contexts where evidence is limited or inconsistent, when primary studies are not feasible due to economic, ethical, or practical constraints, or when clinical and nursing settings present significant logistical challenges [6]

The fundamental distinction between clinical consensus statements (CCSs) and clinical practice guidelines (CPGs) has been thoroughly outlined by Rosenfeld [2]. While CPGs derive their strength from systematic reviews and randomized controlled trials, CCSs are primarily composed of expert opinions grounded in individual experience and knowledge. In this sense, CCSs are particularly valuable in contexts where the available evidence is insufficient to support the development of formal guidelines, yet considerable variability in clinical practice and opportunities for quality improvement persist. Within this framework, efforts to establish standardized approaches for managing cases lacking precise guidelines are gaining increasing relevance, especially in the era of personalized medicine, where clinicians must determine the most appropriate treatment for each patient while safeguarding their unique individuality.

In our review, which aimed to evaluate the rigor of Delphi-method consensuses within the framework of personalized medicine, we began with one of the pioneering approaches: Rosenfeld's method. Although only 22 of the 86 articles included in our analysis explicitly adopted it, Rosenfeld's framework remains the most standardized and consolidated methodology currently available for Delphi consensus. Endorsed by the American Academy of Otolaryngology–Head and Neck Surgery Foundation, it clearly defines key elements such as expert panel selection, questionnaire design, number of rounds, consensus thresholds, and reporting standards. This structured approach has been widely adopted in otolaryngology and other specialties, ensuring greater methodological rigor, transparency, and reproducibility compared with earlier, less formalized strategies. For these reasons, we selected it as the reference model to assess whether the articles adhered to specific methodological criteria.

The second step of our assessment concerned the application of the methodology proposed by Nasa et al. [7]. This framework introduces nine key evaluation domains—including problem identification, expert panel selection, anonymity, iterative rounds, consensus and closing criteria, and response stability—specifically designed to address the frequent methodological inconsistencies observed in Delphi studies. By structuring the process in this way, the approach improves transparency, reproducibility, and overall credibility, making it a valuable tool for both researchers and reviewers in the application of the DeMet to healthcare research.

In our review, only 9 out of 86 studies (10.5%) met enough reliability criteria to be evaluated as "good" [10–19]. This result highlights the widespread methodological weaknesses affecting Delphi studies in healthcare. Recurrent issues included unclear reporting of panel selection, absence of predefined consensus thresholds, arbitrary closing criteria, and insufficient evaluation of response stability. These shortcomings introduce a substantial risk of bias and compromise the transparency, reproducibility, and overall credibility of the consensus process.

Overall, the key methodological challenges we identified include the following:

- Unclear or incomplete panel selection, often preventing assessment of the adequacy and balance of expertise;
- Absence of predefined consensus thresholds, with criteria sometimes introduced post hoc or without explicit justification;
- Arbitrary or undefined closing criteria, leading to uncertainty about when the Delphi process should conclude;
- Lack of evaluation of response stability, making it difficult to verify whether a genuine consensus was achieved.

Finally, we applied the DELPHISTAR criteria to all 86 articles included in our review. This methodology allows an assessment of adherence to its 38-item checklist and highlights critical gaps that may compromise the reproducibility and reliability of Delphi studies in otorhinolaryngology. We observed that some articles showed relatively high compliance with the checklist, such as Craig et al. [10], who adhered to 26 criteria, and Tucci et al. [20], with 25 criteria. Conversely, other studies demonstrated poor adherence, meeting as few as 8 criteria [20,21].

This review has several limitations that should be acknowledged. First, although we adopted a comprehensive search strategy across multiple databases and languages, it is possible that relevant Delphi-based studies in otolaryngology were missing, particularly grey literature, conference proceedings, or studies published in less common languages. Moreover, we restricted our analysis to fully published articles, which may have introduced a publication bias, as studies with less rigorous methods might remain unpublished.

Second, our evaluation was inherently dependent on what was reported in the articles. We cannot exclude that some studies applied more rigorous methodological procedures but failed to describe them adequately in the manuscript. This limitation underscores the very issue our review highlights: incomplete reporting may underestimate the true quality of Delphi studies while simultaneously diminishing their reproducibility, comparability, and impact. Finally, although we applied three established methodological frameworks [2,6,7], these instruments themselves are evolving, and different evaluative criteria might have yielded partially different classifications.

When we state that an article fails to report key elements or displays a high risk of bias, we are not necessarily implying that the research is poor or the scientific work is inadequate. More often, these are outstanding and ambitious studies that suffer only from methodological or reporting shortcomings. Yet, such omissions inevitably narrow their scope and applicability, limiting the impact of what could otherwise be invaluable contributions to the field. Too often, brilliant efforts risk being overshadowed simply because they lack methodological clarity or fail to adhere to standardized frameworks.

For this reason, we believe it is imperative that all researchers in otolaryngology—and beyond—fully embrace established methodological and reporting schemes. Order generates order: adopting standardized frameworks such as Rosenfeld's approach, Nasa's bias domains, and the DELPHISTAR checklist ensures that consensus statements are not only expert-driven but also methodologically sound, transparent, and reproducible. In Delphi-based research, methodology represents not a secondary aspect but the true core of validity—more decisive than the evidence base itself, and even more foundational than expertise. Only through methodological rigor can these studies realize their full potential and continue to shape the future of personalized medicine.

5. Conclusions

This systematic review highlights both the growing role and the persistent methodological challenges of Delphi studies in otorhinolaryngology. Despite their increasing use as tools to guide clinical decision-making in areas where high-level evidence is lacking, the overall methodological rigor remains limited, with only a minority of studies meeting established quality criteria. The methodological frameworks proposed by Rosenfeld et al. [2] and Nasa et al. [7]., together with the recent DELPHISTAR reporting guidelines, provide valuable instruments to enhance transparency, reproducibility, and reliability. However, their partial and inconsistent adoption underscores the urgent need for more rigorous standardization. Enhancing methodological quality is essential not only to improve the reliability of Delphi-derived consensus statements but also to ensure their meaningful integration into the paradigm of personalized medicine, where individualized yet consistent care for each patient remains the ultimate goal.

Supplementary Materials: The following supporting information can be downloaded at https://www.mdpi.com/article/10.3390/jpm15120567/s1. Table S1: PRISMA Checklist; Table S2: List of DeMet consensus articles included and analyzed in this systematic review.

Author Contributions: Conceptualization, A.M.S. methodology, A.M.S., A.U. and G.P.; validation, J.R.L. and A.M.; formal analysis, A.M.S.; investigation, E.B., M.C., M.G.C., B.D., A.L. and L.M.; data curation, E.B., M.C., M.G.C., B.D., A.L. and L.M.; writing—original draft preparation, A.U. and G.P.; writing—review and editing, A.M.S., J.R.L. and A.M.; visualization, G.P.; supervision, A.M.S. All authors have read and agreed to the published version of the manuscript.

Funding: This research received no external funding.

Institutional Review Board Statement: Not applicable.

Informed Consent Statement: Not applicable.

Data Availability Statement: The original contributions presented in this study are included in the article/Supplementary Materials. Further inquiries can be directed to the corresponding author.

Conflicts of Interest: The authors declare no conflicts of interest.

Abbreviations

The following abbreviations are used in this manuscript:

DeMet	Delphi Method

References

1. Khodyakov, D.; Grant, S.; Kroger, J.; Gadwah-Meaden, C.; Motala, A.; Larkin, J. Disciplinary trends in the use of the Del method: A bibliometric analysis. *PLoS ONE* **2023**, *18*, e0289009. [CrossRef] [PubMed]
2. Rosenfeld, R.M.; Nnacheta, L.C.; Corrigan, M.D. Clinical Consensus Statement Development Manual. *Otolaryngol. Neck S* **2015**, *153*, S1–S14. [CrossRef] [PubMed]
3. Hart, L.M.; Jorm, A.F.; Kanowski, L.G.; Kelly, C.M.; Langlands, R.L. Mental health first aid for Indigenous Australians: U Delphi consensus studies to develop guidelines for culturally appropriate responses to mental health problems. *BMC Psychi* **2009**, *9*, 47. [CrossRef] [PubMed]
4. Jünger, S.; Payne, S.A.; Brine, J.; Radbruch, L.; Brearley, S.G. Guidance on Conducting and REporting DElphi Studies (CRED in palliative care: Recommendations based on a methodological systematic review. *Palliat. Med.* **2017**, *31*, 684–706. [CrossRe
5. Gattrell, W.T.; Hungin, A.P.; Price, A.; Winchester, C.C.; Tovey, D.; Hughes, E.L.; van Zuuren, E.J.; Goldman, K.; Logullo Matheis, R.; et al. ACCORD guideline for reporting consensus-based methods in biomedical research and clinical practic study protocol. *Res. Integr. Peer Rev.* **2022**, *7*, 3. [CrossRef] [PubMed]
6. Niederberger, M.; Schifano, J.; Deckert, S.; Hirt, J.; Homberg, A.; Köberich, S.; Kuhn, R.; Rommel, A.; Sonnberger, M.; Network, Delphi studies in social and health sciences—Recommendations for an interdisciplinary standardized reporting (DELPHIST Results of a Delphi study. *PLoS ONE* **2024**, *19*, e0304651. [CrossRef] [PubMed]
7. Nasa, P.; Jain, R.; Juneja, D. Delphi methodology in healthcare research: How to decide its appropriateness. *World, J. Metho* **2021**, *11*, 116–129. [CrossRef] [PubMed]
8. Saibene, A.M. Systematic Review Protocol. OSF. Available online: http://osf.io/8cxs7 (accessed on 18 September 2025).
9. Liberati, A.; Altman, D.G.; Tetzlaff, J.; Mulrow, C.; Gøtzsche, P.C.; Ioannidis, J.P.; Clarke, M.; Devereaux, P.J.; Kleijnen, J.; Mohe The PRISMA statement for reporting systematic reviews and meta-analyses of studies that evaluate healthcare interventi Explanation and elaboration. *J. Clin. Epidemiol.* **2009**, *62*, e1–e34. [CrossRef] [PubMed]
10. Craig, J.R.; Poetker, D.M.; Aksoy, U.; Allevi, F.; Biglioli, F.; Cha, B.Y.; Chiapasco, M.; Lechien, J.R.; Safadi, A.; Dds, R.S.; e Diagnosing odontogenic sinusitis: An international multidisciplinary consensus statement. *Int. Forum Allergy Rhinol.* **2021**, 1235–1248. [CrossRef] [PubMed]
11. Speyer, R.; Balaguer, M.; Cugy, E.; Devoucoux, C.; Morinière, S.; Soriano, G.; Vérin, E.; Woisard, V. Expert Consensus on Clin Decision Making in the Disease Trajectory of Oropharyngeal Dysphagia in Adults: An International Delphi Study. *J. Clin. N* **2023**, *12*, 6572. [CrossRef] [PubMed]

Scharpf, J.; Liu, J.C.; Sinclair, C.; Singer, M.; Liddy, W.; Orloff, L.; Steward, D.; Velez, J.B.; Randolph, G.W. Critical Review and Consensus Statement for Neural Monitoring in Otolaryngologic Head, Neck, and Endocrine Surgery. *Otolaryngol. Neck Surg.* **2021**, *166*, 233–248. [CrossRef] [PubMed]
Saibene, A.M.; Allevi, F.; Ayad, T.; Baudoin, T.; Bernal-Sprekelsen, M.; Briganti, G.; Carrie, S.; Cayé-Thomasen, P.; Saidi, S.D.; Dauby, N.; et al. Appropriateness for SARS-CoV-2 vaccination for otolaryngologist and head and neck surgeons in case of pregnancy, breastfeeding, or childbearing potential: Yo-IFOS and CEORL-HNS joint clinical consensus statement. *Eur. Arch. Oto-Rhino-Laryngol.* **2021**, *278*, 4091–4099. [CrossRef] [PubMed]
Saibene, A.M.; Allevi, F.; Calvo-Henriquez, C.; Dauby, N.; Dondossola, D.; Hervochon, R.; Lechien, J.R.; Lobo-Duro, D.; Locatello, L.G.; Maniaci, A.; et al. Comprehensive management of paranasal sinus fungus balls: A Young-IFOS consensus statement. *Int. Forum Allergy Rhinol.* **2022**, *13*, 877–885. [CrossRef] [PubMed]
Schiff, E.; Propst, E.J.; Balakrishnan, K.; Johnson, K.; Lounsbury, D.W.; Brenner, M.J.; Tawfik, M.; Workgroup, P.T.E.R.; Yang, C.J. Pediatric Tracheostomy Emergency Readiness Assessment Tool: International Consensus Recommendations. *Laryngoscope* **2023**, *133*, 3588–3601. [CrossRef] [PubMed]
Mehanna, H.; Hardman, J.C.; Shenson, J.A.; Abou-Foul, A.K.; Topf, M.C.; AlFalasi, M.; Chan, J.Y.K.; Chaturvedi, P.; Chow, V.L.Y.; Dietz, A.; et al. Recommendations for head and neck surgical oncology practice in a setting of acute severe resource constraint during the COVID-19 pandemic: An international consensus. *Lancet Oncol.* **2020**, *21*, e350–e359. [CrossRef] [PubMed]
Lechien, J.R.; Geneid, A.; Bohlender, J.E.; Cantarella, G.; Avellaneda, J.C.; Desuter, G.; Sjogren, E.V.; Finck, C.; Hans, S.; Hess, M.; et al. Consensus for voice quality assessment in clinical practice: Guidelines of the European Laryngological Society and Union of the European Phoniatricians. *Eur. Arch. Oto-Rhino-Laryngol.* **2023**, *280*, 5459–5473. [CrossRef] [PubMed]
Baudouin, R.; Hans, S.; Guiche, M.; Binet, A.; Circiu, M.P.; Crevier-Buchman, L.; Morsomme, D.; Finck, C.; Rutigliano, P.; Rodriguez, A.; et al. Tele-rehabilitation in voice disorders during the pandemic: A consensus paper from the French Society of Phoniatrics and Laryngology. *Eur. Arch. Oto-Rhino-Laryngol.* **2022**, *280*, 2411–2419. [CrossRef] [PubMed]
Tucci, D.L.; McCoul, E.D.; Rosenfeld, R.M.; Tunkel, D.E.; Batra, P.S.; Chandrasekhar, S.S.; Cordes, S.R.; Eshraghi, A.A.; Kaylie, D.; Lal, D.; et al. Clinical Consensus Statement: Balloon Dilation of the Eustachian Tube. *Otolaryngol. Neck Surg.* **2019**, *161*, 6–17. [CrossRef] [PubMed]
Park, J.-O.; Kim, J.H.; Joo, Y.H.; Kim, S.-Y.; Kim, G.-J.; Kim, H.B.; Hong, H.J.; Park, Y.M.; Chung, E.-J.; Ji, Y.B.; et al. Guideline for the Surgical Management of Locally Invasive Differentiated Thyroid Cancer From the Korean Society of Head and Neck Surgery. *Clin. Exp. Otorhinolaryngol.* **2023**, *16*, 1–19. [CrossRef] [PubMed]
Stack, B.C.; Twining, C.; Rastatter, J.; Angelos, P.; Baloch, Z.; Diercks, G.; Faquin, W.; Kazahaya, K.; Rivkees, S.; Sheyn, T.; et al. Consensus statement by the American Association of Clinical Endocrinology (AACE) and the American Head and Neck Society Endocrine Surgery Section (AHNS-ES) on Pediatric Benign and Malignant Thyroid Surgery. *Head Neck* **2021**, *43*, 1027–1042. [CrossRef] [PubMed]

Journal of
Personalized Medicine

MDPI

Article

Towards a Personalized Vestibular Assessment in Older Patients with Cochlear Implant

Tiziana Di Cesare [1], Pasqualina Maria Picciotti [2,3,*], Walter Di Nardo [2,3], Daniela Rodolico [3] and Jacopo Galli [2,3]

1 Audiology and ENT, Institute for Maternal and Child Health—IRCCS "Burlo Garofolo", 34137 Trieste, Italy; tiziana.dicesare@burlo.trieste.it

2 Department of Head, Neck and Sensory Organs, Università Cattolica del Sacro Cuore, 00168 Rome, Italy; walter.dinardo@policlinicogemelli.it (W.D.N.); jacopo.galli@policlinicogemelli.it (J.G.)

3 Unit of Otorhinolaryngology and Head-Neck Surgery, Fondazione Policlinico Universitario A. Gemelli IRCCS, 00168 Rome, Italy

* Correspondence: pasqualinamaria.picciotti@unicatt.it; Tel.: +39-0630154439

Abstract

Background: Age-related vestibular decline frequently accompanies presbycusis, and older adults undergoing cochlear implantation (CI) may be particularly vulnerable to postoperative dizziness due to a reduced compensatory capacity and a higher burden of comorbidities. Although CI is an effective treatment for severe-to-profound sensorineural hearing loss in the elderly, its impact on vestibular function remains a critical concern. This study aimed to compare pre and postoperative vestibular performance in older patients (≥65 years) versus younger adults undergoing CI in order to identify the risk factors for postoperative vestibular deterioration and critical issues that characterize this category and carry out personalized preoperative counseling. **Methods**: In this monocentric observational study, adults undergoing CI were divided into two groups: older patients (OPS, ≥65 years) and younger patients (YPS, <65 years). Vestibular function was assessed preoperatively and one month postoperatively through a Dizziness Handicap Inventory (DHI), history of recurrent falls, clinical examination, video head impulse test (VHIT), bithermal caloric testing, and computerized dynamic posturography (Sensory Organization Test, SOT). Risk factors for postoperative vestibular worsening were analyzed using ANOVA test and chi-square statistics, with significance set at $p < 0.05$. **Results**: A total of 63 patients were included, with 18 surgeries involving OPS and 45 involving YPS. Preoperatively, OPS showed significantly higher rates of vestibular abnormalities on caloric testing (55.5% vs. 17.7% bilateral hyporeflexia, $p < 0.05$) and a higher prevalence of recurrent falls (33.3% vs. 4.4%, $p < 0.05$). Early postoperative dizziness (DHI^1) increased significantly in both groups, but age ≥ 65 was a risk factor for ≥10% worsening (OR 2.2, $p < 0.05$). At one month, YPS returned to baseline DHI values, whereas OPS showed persistent dizziness with significantly higher DHI^2 scores (29.2 vs. 12.9, $p < 0.05$). Vestibular worsening was identified in 33.3% of VHIT assessments and 44.4% of caloric tests in OPS, with caloric testing proving more sensitive than VHIT. Implantation on the better-functioning vestibular side and the presence of ≥3 comorbidities increased the likelihood of persistent postoperative dizziness. **Conclusions**: Older age is a significant risk factor for persistent dizziness and vestibular impairment one month after CI. Given the reduced compensatory capacity typical of older adults, vestibular assessment should play a central role in preoperative decision-making, particularly for side selection. Bithermal caloric stimulation is recommended as the most sensitive tool for detecting clinically relevant vestibular changes. Preoperative counseling for older CI candidates should include a detailed discussion of vestibular risks and the possible need for postoperative rehabilitation.

Keywords: cochlear implant; vestibular function; older patients; elderly; personalized preoperative cochlear implant counseling

1. Introduction

Hearing rehabilitation in the elderly has undergone significant changes in recent years due to the ever-increasing spread of the problem and the reliability of new cochlear implant (CI) technologies. In fact, it has been estimated that by age 65, a third of people will have enough irreversible damage to hair cells in their inner ear to experience some degree of hearing loss (HL), causing nearly 226 million people over 65 worldwide to suffer from disabling HL who will require hearing rehabilitation [1,2]. This number is projected to double by 2050 considering the actual demographic transition towards an increasingly aging population [2].

The significant improvement of hearing performance in terms of speech recognition outcomes with CI among elderly patients with severe or profound HL, compared with the younger counterparts [3,4], has progressively raised the age of eligibility for surgery to the point of no longer considering it a limitation [5].

Several studies investigating the relationship between age and CI outcomes [5–7] highlight the importance of vestibular function in this population. Vestibular hypofunction is more frequently observed in CI candidates than in age-matched controls [7–9], and age-related factors may influence postoperative balance responses. This is particularly relevant given the close anatomical and physiological relationship between the auditory and vestibular systems, which are often affected by the same degenerative processes. Presbycusis—a progressive auditory impairment not attributable to otologic disease, ototoxic agents, or hereditary conditions—is associated with damage to hair cells, spiral ganglion neurons, and the stria vascularis [1,10]. In parallel, recent studies have focused on age-related vestibular changes and their impact on balance control [11,12]. Chronic dizziness affects almost 30% of individuals over 60 [13], prompting the Bárány Society to introduce the term presbyvestibulopathy to describe older patients with mild bilateral vestibular deficits and symptoms of imbalance or falls [14].

Age-related decline in multisensory integration, impaired visual function, polyneuropathy, central neurological conditions, and sarcopenia may further reduce postural stability and contribute to dizziness in the elderly [15]. Notably, dizziness is a common postoperative symptom—often influenced by anesthetic factors—particularly in older patients.

The aim of the present study was to evaluate the vestibular function before and after cochlear implantation in older patients, analyzing the impact of CI surgery on the vestibular system and the role of vestibular assessment compared to younger counterparts. Results could make clinicians aware of the risk factors for postoperative vestibular deterioration and critical issues that characterize this category in order to carry out personalized preoperative counseling.

2. Materials and Methods

It was a monocentric observational study approved by the Ethical Committee of Foundation Polyclinic University A. Gemelli IRCCS, Rome, Italy (protocol code 0012424/23; date of approval 13 April 2023). We included adult (>18 years) CI candidates affected by severe-to-profound SNHL. They were divided in two groups: the older patients (OPS) $\geq$ 65 years old and the younger patients (YPS) < 65 years old.

https://doi.org/10.3390/jpm16020081

The surgical approach was conservative with the intracochlear placement of the array through the (extended) round window membrane except in the case of ossification, when the cochleostomy technique was performed. All patients had sufficient ability to read, understand, and complete the assigned questionnaires and sign an informed consent form. We included CIs of all brands.

Bilateral simultaneous implantations were excluded from the study; in case of bilateral sequential implantations, we considered only the first CI surgery. Bilateral sequential implantations with an interval time < 1 month between the two surgeries were also excluded. History of vestibular schwannoma, active middle ear disease, and congenital malformations of the auditory/vestibular system were exclusion criteria.

General history included a detailed interview about comorbidities, considering hypertension, ischemic heart disease, anxious–depressive syndromes, autoimmune disease, osteoporosis, thyroid disease, diabetes, epilepsy or other neurological disorders, oncological problems, and other diseases.

Vestibular Evaluation

- The Dizziness Handicap Inventory (DHI) (Italian version by Nola et al. [16]) was administered 24–48 h before surgery (DHI^0), 24–48 h after surgery (DHI^1), and one month after surgery (before CI activation) (DHI^2) to evaluate the pre, peri, and postoperative dizziness, respectively [9,16]. It consists of 25 multiple choice questions ("yes"—4 points, "sometimes"—2 points, and "no"—0 points), which provide a total score from 0 (no handicaps) to 100 (the greatest ailment imaginable). Values are considered normal (<10), borderlines (10–16), mild (18–34), moderate (36–52), and severe (≥54).
- Recurrent falls: Each patient was interviewed regarding the presence of recurrent falls in their daily life, providing a choice of 3 answers: "yes" (4 points), "sometimes" (2 points), and "no" (0 points).
- Vestibular assessment was performed 24–48 h before surgery and one month after surgery (before CI activation), including:
    - Clinical examination to assess the presence of spontaneous and/or positional nystagmus and to perform the head-shaking test (HST) and clinical head impulse test (HIT).
    - Video head impulse test (VHIT) using a VOG device (ICS Impulse, GN Otometrics, Taastrup, Denmark) to measure the gain of VOR (Vestibular–Oculomotor Reflex) for both the horizontal canals. It was performed with the patient sitting upright and fixating a visual target in front of him when the clinician generated head impulses by moving it abruptly and unpredictably in the horizontal plane. We considered normal VOR gain > 0.8 and normal gain asymmetry < 20% [9,17].
    - Bitermic caloric stimulation by the Fitzgerald–Hallpike technique (ICS Aircal Air Caloric Sprinkler Otometrics, Taastrup, Denmark). It was performed in a conventional manner (air-flow of 0.8 L/min at temperatures of 50 °C and 24 °C for 60 s, in the dark, in supine position with the head raised at 30°). Nystagmus amplitude was calculated by the system as slow phase velocity (SPV) and measured in °/s. The Jongkee's formula was used to quantify the asymmetry between the sides. Results were expressed as unilateral weakness (UW normal < 15%) and directional preponderance degree (DP normal < 15%). Bilateral hyporeflexia was defined by the sum of the maximal peak velocities of the slow phase caloric-induced nystagmus for stimulation with warm and cold water on each side (SPV) < 25°/s [9,18].

https://doi.org/10.3390/jpm1602C

- Computed Dynamic Posturography (CDP) (Equitest, Neurocom Int. Inc., Clackamas, OR, USA) was performed with the patient standing on a dual footplate enclosed by a visual surround in six balance conditions (eyes open/closed; visual surround steady/rotated; platform steady/rotated—Sensory Organization Test (SOT)) as previously described [19]. For each test, we considered the Composite Equilibrium Score (CES) showing the weighted average of the different conditions and Sensory Analysis (SA) showing the contribution of the different sensorial afferences (somatosensory, visual, vestibular, and visual-preference). We considered normal CES and SA to be >70 [9,19].

3. Statistical Analysis

The sample was described in its clinical and demographic characteristics using descriptive statistics techniques. Continuous values with normal distribution, such as VOR gain and percentage of asymmetry on VHIT, were expressed as mean ± standard deviation (SD). Qualitative variables were expressed as absolute and relative percentages.

The ANOVA test was used to compare the mean scores of the DHI questionnaire, recurrent falls, VHIT, caloric test, and SOT before and after surgery in the two groups (older and younger patients).

The chi-square test (χ^2 test and the odds ratios (OR) with 95% confidence intervals) was used to identify anamnestic and surgical risk factors for postoperative vestibular damage. For the purpose of the study, we considered as MCID (Minimal Clinically Important Difference) any value $\geq$ 10% (DHI, VOR gain on the implanted side, SPV nystagmus on the implanted side, and CES) after surgery compared to the starting score (for example, if a patient had a total preoperative DHI score of 50, any increment $\geq$ 5 points was considered significant). The choice to consider the MCDI as a percentage value and not as a fixed numerical value was dictated by the desire of the authors of the present manuscript to adapt the significance of the worsening score to the starting value of each patient [9]. The results were considered statistically significant for $p < 0.05$.

4. Results

We included 63 patients (36 F, 27 M; mean age 51.4 ± 15.6, range 18–84 years) with a complete vestibular assessment before and after.

Older patients (OPS) were 18 (10 F, 12 M; mean age 70.6 ± 15.9, range 65–84 years).

Causes of deafness were as follows: one genetic 5% (MELAS); one autoimmune cerebellar ataxia (5%); one viral infection 5% (one herpes zoster); one otosclerosis (5%); two drug ototoxicity (10.5%); three Meniere's disease (15.8%); four Sudden Sensorineural Hearing Loss (25%); five presbycusis (25%).

They suffered from, on average, 2.5 comorbidities (range 0–6): 15 (83.3%) were affected by hypertension; 5 (27.7%) by ischemic heart disease; 3 by (16.6%) anxious–depressive syndromes; 4 (22.2%) by autoimmune disease; 1 (5.5%) by osteoporosis; 2 (11.1%) by thyroid disease; 7 (38.8%) by diabetes; 2 (11.1%) by epilepsy or other neurological diseases; 2 by (11.1%) oncological disease; 11 (61.1%) by other nonspecific diseases.

The younger group (YPS) included 45 patients (27 F, 18 M; men age 43.7 ± 15.8, range 18–64).

Their causes of deafness were genetic in 12 patients (26.6%) (9 related to connexin26 mutation and 3 syndromic, 1 Cogan, 1 Epstein, 1 Waardenburg); traumatic in 3 (6.6%) (1 electrocution and 2 temporal bone fractures); 1 (2.2%) meningitis; 4 (8.8%) otosclerosis; 1 (2.2%) chronic cholesteatomatous otitis media; 1 (2.2%) drug ototoxicity; 4 (8.8%) viral infections (1 cytomegalovirus; 1 paramyxovirus; 2 herpes zoster); 1 (2.2%) Sudden Sensorineural Hearing Loss; 18 (40%) idiopathic.

https://doi.org/10.3390/jpm16020081

In regard to comorbidities, younger patients suffered from 0.95 disease, which was statistically lower than the elderly ($p < 0.05$). Seven (15.5%) were affected by hypertension; one (2%) by ischemic heart disease; six (13.3%) by anxious–depressive syndromes; three (6.6%) by autoimmune disease; three (6.6%) by osteoporosis; four (8.8%) by thyroid disease; four (8.8%) by diabetes; six (13.3%) by epilepsy or other neurological diseases; one (2.2%) by oncological disease; five (11.1%) by other nonspecific diseases.

The 100% (18/18) OPS vs. the 51% (23/45) YPS suffered from at least 1 disease ($p < 0.05$), the 39% (7/18) vs. the 22% (10/45) 2–3 comorbidities ($p < 0.05$), and the 39% (7/18) vs. the 4.5% (2/45) had >3 comorbidities ($p < 0.05$).

The preoperative vestibular evaluation showed no significant difference for the mean values of DHI between the younger and the older populations (13.4 vs. 19, $p > 0.05$). In any case, 16/45 (35.5%) younger patients reported abnormal values of DHI^0 compared to the 50% (9/18) of the older patients ($p < 0.05$) (Figure 1).

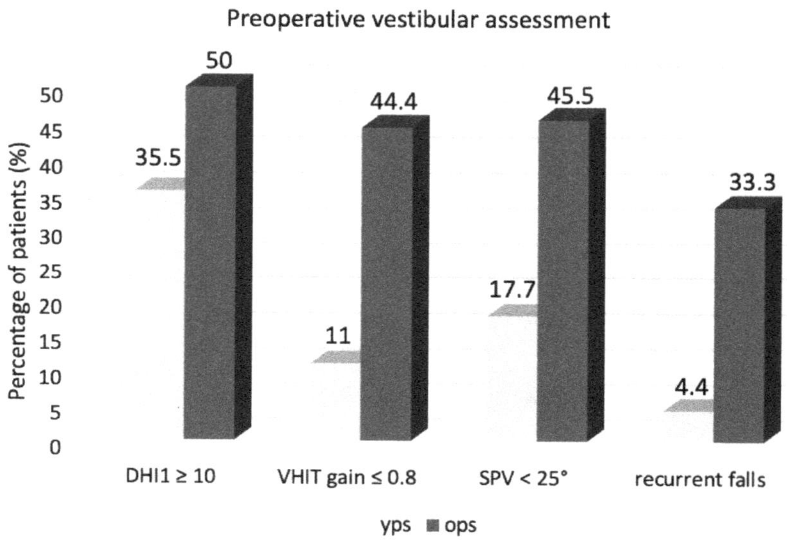

Figure 1. Preoperative vestibular assessment in younger (YPS) and older patients (OPS). DHI0: preoperative Dizziness Handicap Inventory; VHIT: video head impulse test; SPV: slow phase caloric-induced nystagmus velocity.

A significant percentage of OPS (6/18, 33.3%) reported a history of recurrent falls compared to the younger counterparts (2/45, 4.4%) ($p < 0.05$) (Figure 1).

Five YPS (11%) had abnormal VOR gain (<0.8) in the side to be implanted; 8/45 (17.7%) had a significant asymmetry between the two sides (Figure 1).

Among the older population, 8/18 (44.4%) had an abnormal VOR gain in the side to be implanted (Figure 1); 7/18 (38.9%) had a bilateral hypofunction measured with the VHIT. Excluding three of them (one with autoimmune cerebellar ataxia and two with Meniere's disease), 4/18 (22.2%) OPS were in accordance with the diagnostic criteria for the presbyvestibulopathy of the Bárány Society [14]. Five (27.7%) OPS had a significant asymmetry of the VOR gain.

The preoperative caloric stimulation showed an abnormal UW In 17/45 (37.7%) YPS compared to 7/18 (38.9%) OPS. Bilateral hyporeflexia (SPV < 25%) resulted in 8/45 (17.7%) YPS and 10/18 OPS (55.5%) ($p < 0.05$) (Figure 1). Consequently, 7/18 (38.9%) older patients met the criteria for the presbyvestibulopathy using the caloric stimulation.

https://doi.org/10.3390/jpm16020

The mean preoperative Composite Equilibrium Score (CES) of the Sensory Organization Test (SOT) was 54 in OPS (85 somatosensory, 35.3 vestibular, 72.5 visual, and 72 visual-preference) and 71 in YPS (92.6 somatosensory, 54.6 vestibular, 72 visual, 87 visual-preference) ($p < 0.05$ for vestibular scores comparison).

The early (24–48 h) postoperative DHI^1 was 23.2 for YPS and 29 for OPS, without a significant difference ($p > 0.05$). In any case, in both groups the early postoperative increase in dizziness perception was significant ($p < 0.05$). The age $\geq$ 65 represented a risk factor for a significant ($\geq$10%) worsening of the DHI 24–48 h after surgery (OR = 2.2; CI = 0.7–6.8; $p < 0.05$) (Figure 2). In both groups, the presence of $\geq$3 comorbidities was a risk factor (OR = 2.05; CI = 0.5–7.7; $p < 0.05$).

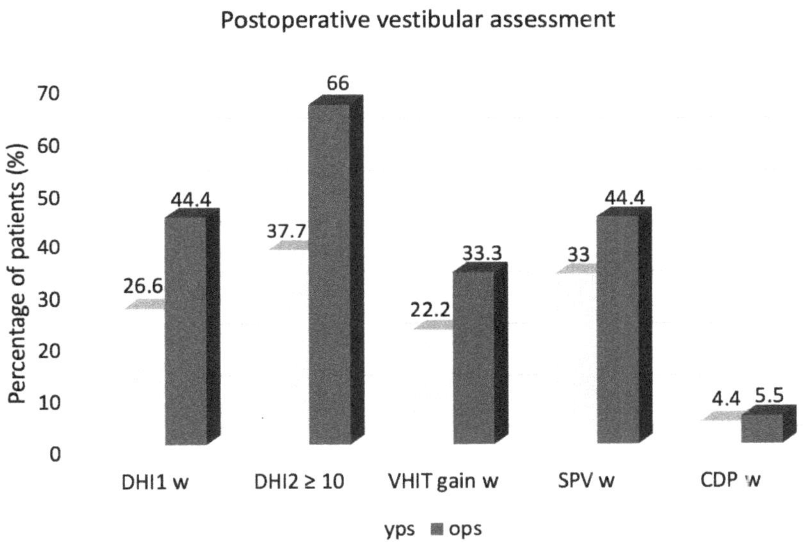

Figure 2. Postoperative vestibular assessment in younger (YPS) and older patients (OPS). DHI1: Dizziness Handicap Inventory 24–48 h; VHIT: video head impulse test; SPV: slow phase caloric-induced nystagmus velocity; w: significant worsening; DHI2: Dizziness Handicap Inventory 1 month.

The late postoperative evaluation showed a significant difference between the two groups for the mean DHI^2 (12.9 vs. 29.2, $p < 0.05$). Consequently, while most young patients showed a decrease in the total score compared to the immediate postoperative period, with no difference between DHI^0 and DHI^2 in this group ($p < 0.05$), most older patients demonstrated a persistence of the dizziness perception 1 month after surgery, with a significant increase compared to the preoperative evaluation ($p > 0.05$). The age $\geq$ 65 years was a risk factor for the presence of dizziness after 1 month (OR = 3.3; CI = 1–10.4; $p < 0.05$) (Figure 2).

In 16/63 cochlear implantations (25.4%), the VHIT showed a significant worsening ($\geq$ 0.1) of the VOR gain in the implanted side after surgery; it involved 6/18 (33.3%) surgeries performed in OPS and 10/45 (22.2%) surgeries performed in the younger population (OR = 1.75; CI = 0.5–5.8; $p < 0.05$) (Figure 2).

The chronic bilateral hypofunction or the diagnosis of presbyvestibulopathy were not related to the worsening after surgery.

In 23/63 ears (36.5%) the caloric test demonstrated a significant worsening of the SPV in the implanted ear after surgery, involving 8/18 (44.4%) surgeries performed in OPS and

https://doi.org/10.3390/jpm16020081

15/45 (33%) in YPS (OR = 1.6; CI = 0.5–4.9; $p < 0.05$) (Figure 2). In both groups, the caloric test was more sensible compared to VHIT.

As for VHIT, the preoperative bilateral vestibular hyporeflexia or the diagnosis of presbyvestibulopathy were not risk factors for a significant reduction in the evoked nystagmus with the caloric test. Among the elderly, Meniere's disease (OR = 4.8; CI = 0.35–65.7; $p < 0.05$) and the presence of ≥ 3 comorbidities (OR = 2.2; CI = 0.2–20.4; $p < 0.05$) were risk factors for vestibular damage.

In both groups, the cochlear implantation in the hyper-functioning side, in case of asymmetry, was related to the persistence of postoperative dizziness after 1 month ($p < 0.05$).

In both groups, the mean postoperative scores of CDP were not different ($p > 0.05$). Only three patients in the total sample (4.7%) demonstrated a significant worsening of the CES, 1/18 (5.5%) in OPS and 2/45 (4.4%) in YPS ($p > 0.05$).

5. Discussion

This study provides a comprehensive evaluation of vestibular function before and after cochlear implantation in adults over 65 years of age, comparing outcomes with a younger cohort. The findings confirm that advanced age is associated with both a higher prevalence of preoperative vestibular dysfunction and a greater likelihood of persistent postoperative dizziness.

Consistent with the previous literature reports, the older cohort in our study presented a significantly higher proportion of vestibular deficits before surgery—both in VHIT and caloric testing—than younger participants. This aligns with current pathophysiological models of presbyvestibulopathy, which describe age-related degeneration affecting hair cells, vestibular nerve fibers, and central pathways involved in balance control, as well as age-related cochlear degeneration (presbycusis) [10–14]. Notably, 44–55% of older patients met diagnostic criteria for presbyvestibulopathy, which is comparable to prevalence estimates reported by the Bárány Society in individuals over 70 years of age [14]. Likewise, the markedly higher incidence of recurrent falls among older adults correlates with prior findings showing that nearly one-third of people over 60 experience chronic dizziness or imbalance, with substantial repercussions for daily function and fall risk [12,13,20]. Lovin et al. [7] have also shown that older cochlear implant candidates are more likely than age-matched controls to present vestibular hypofunction, supporting the hypothesis of shared vulnerability between auditory and vestibular structures. The significantly higher burden of comorbidities in the older group—many of which interfere with multisensory integration and motor control—further contributes to this predisposition.

Regarding our vestibular findings after CI, both age groups reported a significant increase in dizziness during the first 24–48 h after surgery, in agreement with the literature [8,9]. However, age $\geq$ 65 years emerged as a clear predictor of greater early postoperative worsening on the Dizziness Handicap Inventory, reflecting a reduced short-term vestibular compensatory capacity in older adults. Indeed, previous research suggests that aging is associated with reduced cerebellar plasticity, slower sensory rebalancing, and reduced postural reserve, all of which may delay early compensatory mechanisms [11,12]. Furthermore, caloric stimulation has been shown to be more sensitive than VHIT in detecting early postoperative vestibular changes, a finding consistent with recent meta-analyses and clinical studies [8,17,18]. This increased sensitivity of caloric testing is particularly relevant in older adults, who often exhibit early deficits in low-frequency vestibular responses, which caloric testing is better suited to detect [12].

On the other hand, the one-month evaluation after CI highlights a highly significant finding regarding the persistence of dizziness in the older cohort, in contrast to the recovery

https://doi.org/10.3390/jpm16020

observed in younger patients. Age ≥ 65 years was a significant independent risk factor for persistent symptoms at one month. We hypothesize that the high prevalence of bilateral vestibular involvement before implantation and comorbidities, including polyneuropathy, visual impairment, metabolic and neurological disorders, and sarcopenia, hinder vestibular compensation. Reduced efficacy of vestibular rehabilitation in older adults has also been described in the literature, supported by neurophysiological evidence [12]. In our study, the presence of more than three comorbidities was associated with early and persistent postoperative dizziness, highlighting the importance of a multidimensional geriatric assessment both before and after CI.

Another important finding of our analysis concerns the side to be implanted. Our data confirm that implantation on the side with better function in cases of preoperative vestibular asymmetry is associated with a higher probability of persistent dizziness, in agreement with previous studies [7,9]. This underlines the clinical relevance of preoperative vestibular testing to guide side selection, particularly in older adults who show slower and less complete compensation.

Based on our results, several clinical implications emerge. The first concerns the need for a comprehensive vestibular evaluation in CI candidates, especially those ≥65 years of age, both to identify presbyvestibulopathy and to guide surgical planning. This evaluation should include the bithermal caloric test, which has demonstrated greater sensitivity than VHIT. The second consideration concerns the general evaluation for possible comorbidities, given their significant contribution to postoperative disequilibrium. The third point concerns the need for preoperative counseling to explicitly address the increased risk of persistent dizziness in older adults, even when a favorable hearing outcome is expected. Patients should also be informed of the possibility of vestibular rehabilitation, which should be strongly recommended to reduce the risk of falls and facilitate recovery.

Finally, we must necessarily state some limitations of the present study, which concern the small number of the sample examined, the absence of an assessment of vestibular potentials (VEMPs), and the lack of a long-term follow-up that would provide a clearer understanding of the temporal course of vestibular compensation.

A further limitation is the lack of assessment of vestibular-evoked myogenic potentials (VEMPs). It is known that the otolithic organs, particularly the saccule, are vulnerable to both age-related degeneration and cochlear implant-related trauma, and isolated otolithic dysfunction can occur even in the presence of preserved semicircular canal function [21–23]. Therefore, vestibular assessment using VHIT and caloric testing may underestimate the extent of vestibular damage in elderly patients. This limitation may be clinically relevant, as otolithic dysfunction can be associated with impaired postural control and an increased risk of falls, especially in the elderly [21,24]. Therefore, the lack of VEMP assessment in our study may have led to an underestimation of fall risk and may partly explain the persistence of dizziness and imbalance observed in elderly patients despite normal canal function.

Future studies should, therefore, include a comprehensive vestibular assessment incorporating otolithic function tests to better characterize vestibular impairment and improve fall risk stratification in elderly cochlear implant candidates.

6. Conclusions

An age over 65 years is a risk factor for the persistence of vertigo symptoms one month after cochlear implant surgery. Considering the potential difficulty of performing vestibular rehabilitation in elderly patients in the postoperative period, the hypofunctioning side should be chosen whenever possible. The preferable test is bithermal caloric stimulation as it is more sensitive than VHIT. Aspects relating to vestibular function of the elderly patient

https://doi.org/10.3390/jpm16020081

should be given attention in the preoperative stage in order to personalize counseling and postoperative treatment.

Author Contributions: Conceptualization, T.D.C. and P.M.P.; methodology, T.D.C. and P.M.P.; software, T.D.C. and D.R.; validation, P.M.P. and J.G.; formal analysis, T.D.C.; investigation, T.D.C. and D.R.; data curation, T.D.C., P.M.P. and D.R.; writing—original draft preparation, T.D.C. and P.M.P.; writing—review and editing, T.D.C., P.M.P., W.D.N. and J.G.; supervision, W.D.N. and J.G.; project administration, P.M.P. and J.G. All authors have read and agreed to the published version of the manuscript.

Funding: This research received no external funding.

Institutional Review Board Statement: The study was conducted in accordance with the Declaration of Helsinki, and approved by the Ethics Committee of Foundation Polyclinic University A. Gemelli IRCCS, Rome, Italy (protocol code 0012424/23; date of approval 13 April 2023).

Informed Consent Statement: Informed consent was obtained from all subjects involved in the study.

Data Availability Statement: The raw data supporting the conclusions of this article will be made available by the authors on request.

Conflicts of Interest: The authors declare no conflicts of interest.

References

1. Wu, P.Z.; O'Malley, J.T.; de Gruttola, V.; Liberman, M.C. Age-Related Hearing Loss Is Dominated by Damage to Inner Ear Sens Cells, Not the Cellular Battery That Powers Them. *J. Neurosci.* **2020**, *40*, 6357–6366. [CrossRef]
2. Chadha, S.; Kamenov, K.; Cieza, A. The world report on hearing, 2021. *Bull. World Health Organ.* **2021**, *99*, 242–242A. [Cross
3. Lally, J.W.; Adams, J.K.; Wilkerson, B.J. The use of cochlear implantation in the elderly. *Curr. Opin. Otolaryngol. Head Neck S* **2019**, *27*, 387–391. [CrossRef]
4. Bourn, S.S.; Goldstein, M.R.; Morris, S.A.; Jacob, A. Cochlear implant outcomes in the very elderly. *Am. J. Otolaryngol.* **2** *43*, 103200. [CrossRef] [PubMed]
5. Rohloff, K.; Koopmann, M.; Wei, D.; Rudack, C.; Savvas, E. Cochlear Implantation in the Elderly: Does Age Matter? *Otol. Neur* **2017**, *38*, 54–59. [CrossRef] [PubMed]
6. Wong, D.J.; Moran, M.; O'Leary, S.J. Outcomes After Cochlear Implantation in the Very Elderly. *Otol. Neurotol.* **2016**, *37*, 46 [CrossRef]
7. Lovin, B.D.; Gorelik, D.; Lin, K.F.; Vrabec, J.T. Vestibular Hypofunction Screening in Older Cochlear Implant Candida *Otolaryngol. Head Neck Surg.* **2024**, *171*, 858–863. [CrossRef]
8. Vaz, F.C.; Petrus, L.; Martins, W.R.; Silva, I.M.C.; Lima, J.A.O.; Santos, N.M.D.S.; Turri-Silva, N.; Bahmad, F., Jr. The effec cochlear implant surgery on vestibular function in adults: A meta-analysis study. *Front. Neurol.* **2022**, *13*, 947589. [Cross [PubMed]
9. Picciotti, P.M.; Di Cesare, T.; Rodolico, D.; Di Nardo, W.; Galli, J. Clinical and Instrumental Evaluation of Vestibular Func Before and After Cochlear Implantation in Adults. *Audiol. Res.* **2025**, *15*, 71. [CrossRef]
10. Zhao, X.; Shen, T.; Cao, S.; Liu, Z.; Pang, W.; Li, M.; Liu, J.; Li, W.; Wu, Y.; Liu, C.; et al. Presbycusis: Pathology, Signal Pathw and Therapeutic Strategy. *Adv. Sci.* **2025**, *12*, e2410413. [CrossRef]
11. Manrique, M.J.; Batuecas, Á.; Cenjor, C.; Ferrán, S.; Gómez, J.R.; Lorenzo, A.I.; Marco, J.; Matiñó, E.; Morant, A.; Morera, C., e Presbycusis and balance disorders in the elderly. Bibliographical review of ethiopathogenic aspects, consequences on qualit life and positive effects of its treatment. *Acta Otorrinolaringol. (Engl. Ed.)* **2023**, *74*, 124–132. [CrossRef]
12. Wagner, A.R.; Akinsola, O.; Chaudhari, A.M.W.; Bigelow, K.E.; Merfeld, D.M. Measuring Vestibular Contributions to Age-Rela Balance Impairment: A Review. *Front. Neurol.* **2021**, *12*, 635305. [CrossRef]
13. Jahn, K. The Aging Vestibular System: Dizziness and Imbalance in the Elderly. *Adv. Otorhinolaryngol.* **2019**, *82*, 143–149. [Cross [PubMed]
14. Agrawal, Y.; Van de Berg, R.; Wuyts, F.; Walther, L.; Magnusson, M.; Oh, E.; Sharpe, M.; Strupp, M. Presbyvestibulopa Diagnostic criteria Consensus document of the classification committee of the Bárány Society. *J. Vestib. Res.* **2019**, *29*, 161– [CrossRef]
15. Iwasaki, S.; Yamasoba, T. Dizziness and Imbalance in the Elderly: Age-related Decline in the Vestibular System. *Aging Dis.* **2** *6*, 38–47. [CrossRef]

https://doi.org/10.3390/jpm1602

Nola, G.; Mostardini, C.; Salvi, C.; Ercolani, A.P.; Ralli, G. Validity of Italian adaptation of the Dizziness Handicap Inventory (DHI) and evaluation of the quality of life in patients with acute dizziness. *Acta Otorhinolaryngol. Ital.* **2010**, *30*, 190. [PubMed]

Picciotti, P.M.; Rolesi, R.; Rossi, G.; Tizio, A.; Sergi, B.; Galli, J. Caloric Test, and Qualitative and Quantitative vHIT Analysis in Vestibular Schwannoma. *Otol. Neurotol.* **2025**, *46*, e215–e223. [CrossRef]

Molnár, A.; Maihoub, S.; Tamás, L.; Szirmai, Á. A possible objective test to detect benign paroxysmal positional vertigo. The role of the caloric and video-head impulse tests in the diagnosis. *J. Otol.* **2022**, *17*, 46–49. [CrossRef] [PubMed]

Picciotti, P.M.; Fiorita, A.; Di Nardo, W.; Quaranta, N.; Paludetti, G.; Maurizi, M. VEMPs and dynamic posturography after intratympanic gentamycin in Menière's disease. *J. Vestib. Res.* **2005**, *15*, 161–168. [CrossRef]

Picciotti, P.M.; Di Cesare, T.; Libonati, F.A.; Libonati, G.A.; Paludetti, G.; Galli, J. Presbycusis and pres-byvestibulopathy: Balance improvement after hearing loss restoration. *Hear. Balance Commun.* **2024**, *22*, 94–99. [CrossRef]

Agrawal, Y.; Merfeld, D.M.; Horak, F.B.; Redfern, M.S.; Manor, B.; Westlake, K.P.; Holstein, G.R.; Smith, P.F.; Bhatt, T.; Bohnen, N.I.; et al. Aging, Vestibular Function, and Balance: Proceedings of a National Institute on Aging/National Institute on Deafness and Other Communication Disorders Workshop. *J. Gerontol. A Biol. Sci. Med. Sci.* **2020**, *75*, 2471–2480. [CrossRef]

Ji, L.; Zhai, S. Aging and the peripheral vestibular system. *J. Otol.* **2018**, *13*, 138–140. [CrossRef] [PubMed]

Ayas, M.; Muzaffar, J.; Phillips, V.; Smith, M.E.; Borsetto, D.; Bance, M.L. Effect of Cochlear Implantation on Air Conduction and Bone Conduction Elicited Vestibular Evoked Myogenic Potentials—A Scoping Review. *J. Clin. Med.* **2024**, *13*, 6996. [CrossRef] [PubMed]

McCaslin, D.L.; Jacobson, G.P.; Grantham, S.L.; Piker, E.G.; Verghese, S. The influence of unilateral saccular impairment on functional balance performance and self-report dizziness. *J. Am. Acad. Audiol.* **2011**, *22*, 542–549. [CrossRef] [PubMed]

https://doi.org/10.3390/jpm16020081

Journal of
Personalized Medicine

Article

The Diagnostic Gap Between Clinical and Pathological Extranodal Extension in Head and Neck Cancers: A 5-Year Nationwide Trend Analysis in Taiwan

Hsuen-Fu Lin [1] and Shih-Han Hung [2,*]

[1] Department of Hematology and Oncology, Mennonite Christian Hospital, Hualien 970, Taiwan; mosqlin@gmail.com
[2] Department of Otolaryngology-Head and Neck Surgery, Mennonite Christian Hospital, Hualien 970, Taiwan
* Correspondence: seedturtle@gmail.com; Tel.: +886-3-824-1234

Abstract

Background: Extranodal extension (ENE) is a critical prognostic factor in head and neck squamous cell carcinoma (HNSCC) and was incorporated into the AJCC eighth-edition staging system. However, the concordance between clinical (cENE) and pathological (pENE) ENE remains poorly understood in real-world practice. **Methods:** We conducted a retrospective analysis using Taiwan Cancer Registry (TCR) long-form data from 2018 to 2022, focusing on four major HNSCC sites (oral cavity, oropharynx, hypopharynx, and larynx). The diagnostic gap was defined as the difference between pENE and cENE positivity rates. **Results:** Among 29,830 patients, a persistent diagnostic gap was observed across all sites: laryngeal (20.8%), hypopharyngeal (20.4%), oropharyngeal (11.5%), and oral cavity (9.9%). For oral cavity cancer, the gap did not narrow over the 5-year period (p = 0.9788). Furthermore, in oral cavity cancer, medical centers demonstrated a larger gap than non-medical centers (10.5% vs. 8.4%), a phenomenon we term the "Quality-Gap Paradox". **Conclusions:** A significant diagnostic gap persists in HNSCC, highlighting the limitations of current imaging. The Quality-Gap Paradox, observed in oral cavity cancer, suggests this is driven by a complex interplay of factors including superior pathological detection in high-volume centers. Our findings underscore the need for advanced, personalized risk-stratification tools to bridge this gap and improve patient management.

Keywords: extranodal extension; head and neck cancer; diagnostic gap; Taiwan Cancer Registry; AJCC eighth edition; personalized medicine

1. Introduction

Extranodal extension (ENE), the invasion of cancer cells through the lymph node capsule into surrounding connective tissue, is one of the most powerful adverse prognostic factors in head and neck squamous cell carcinoma (HNSCC) [1,2]. Its presence is associated with a significant increase in the risk of distant metastasis and a decrease in overall survival, often halving a patient's prognosis [3]. Recognizing its profound impact, the American Joint Committee on Cancer (AJCC) incorporated ENE into the eighth-edition staging system for HNSCC, upstaging any ENE-positive node to the N3b category, regardless of size or number [4].

However, the clinical implementation of this staging criterion is hampered by a significant challenge: the diagnostic gap between clinical ENE (cENE), detected preoperatively by imaging modalities like computed tomography (CT) and magnetic resonance imaging (MRI), and pathological ENE (pENE), the gold standard confirmed by postoperative histopathological examination. Systematic reviews have consistently shown that the sensitivity of imaging for detecting ENE is suboptimal, often hovering around 60–70% [5,6]. This means a substantial proportion of patients with microscopic ENE (mENE) are not identified before surgery, leading to potential under-staging and under-treatment.

This issue is particularly relevant in Taiwan, where oral cavity cancer is a major public health concern, largely driven by the widespread practice of betel quid chewing [7,8]. The high incidence provides a unique opportunity to study the real-world implications of the AJCC eighth edition on a large, nationwide scale. To our knowledge, no large-scale study has evaluated the trend of the cENE-pENE diagnostic gap in Taiwan since the implementation of the new staging system. Understanding the magnitude, trend, and contributing factors of this gap is crucial for improving diagnostic accuracy, refining treatment strategies, and advancing personalized medicine in HNSCC.

This study aims to conduct a comprehensive, nationwide analysis of the diagnostic gap between cENE and pENE in four major HNSCC sites (oral cavity, oropharynx, hypopharynx, and larynx) using data from the Taiwan Cancer Registry (TCR) from 2018 to 2022. We hypothesize that a significant diagnostic gap persists and has not narrowed over time. We will also investigate the "Quality-Gap Paradox"—the counterintuitive hypothesis that higher-quality medical centers may exhibit a larger gap due to more meticulous pathological examination.

2. Materials and Methods

2.1. Data Source and Study Population

This retrospective cohort study utilized data from the Taiwan Cancer Registry (TCR) long-form database, a mandatory, population-based cancer registry covering over 98% of all cancer cases in Taiwan. We included all patients newly diagnosed with squamous cell carcinoma of the oral cavity, oropharynx, hypopharynx, and larynx between 1 January 2018, and 31 December 2022. This period was chosen to coincide with the implementation of the AJCC 8th edition, ensuring consistent ENE definitions. Patients with distant metastasis at diagnosis (M1), unknown ENE status, or those who did not undergo neck dissection were excluded from the pENE analysis.

2.2. Variable Definitions

Site-Specific Factors (SSF) in the TCR are standardized codes used to capture detailed, cancer-specific information not included in general staging. For HNSCC, SSF9 and SSF10 are used to document ENE status.

Clinical ENE (cENE): Defined based on SSF9. A case was considered cENE-positive if the code was 010, 020, or 030. These codes correspond to clinical or radiographic evidence of ENE based on imaging findings such as ill-defined nodal borders, infiltration into adjacent fat or muscle, or frank invasion of nearby structures, consistent with recently standardized international criteria [9,10]. The cENE rate was the number of cENE-positive cases divided by the total number of cases with a valid SSF9 entry.

Pathological ENE (pENE): Defined based on SSF10. A case was considered pENE-positive if the code was 010, 020, or 030. These codes indicate pathologically confirmed ENE, defined as tumor extension through the lymph node capsule into the surrounding perinodal soft tissue, as identified by histopathological examination. The pENE rate was the number of pENE-positive cases divided by the total number of cases that underwent neck dissection.

Hospital Level: In Taiwan, hospitals are officially accredited by the Ministry of Health and Welfare into different tiers. Medical centers represent the highest tier, equivalent to tertiary care or academic medical centers in other healthcare systems. These institutions are

https://doi.org/10.3390/jpm16020123

required to meet stringent criteria, including: (1) provision of comprehensive subspecialty services across all major disciplines; (2) maintenance of advanced diagnostic and therapeutic technologies; (3) active involvement in medical education and training programs; and (4) demonstrated capacity for high-volume, complex case management. Non-medical centers include regional hospitals (comparable to secondary care hospitals) and district hospitals, which provide general and some specialized services but may not have the full range of subspecialties or the same research and teaching infrastructure. For this study, hospitals were categorized as medical centers or non-medical centers based on the official accreditation status provided by the TCR at the time of patient diagnosis.

Diagnostic Gap: The primary outcome, calculated as the absolute difference between the pENE rate and the cENE rate (Gap = pENE% − cENE%). It is important to note that the diagnostic gap, as defined here, is a population-level metric that quantifies the overall under-detection of ENE by clinical/imaging assessment relative to pathological examination. It does not represent individual-patient concordance or discordance, nor does it directly measure the sensitivity or specificity of clinical ENE detection, which would require patient-level paired cENE and pENE data. Rather, the gap reflects the aggregate difference in detection rates across the population and serves as an indicator of the clinical challenge in preoperatively identifying ENE.

2.3. *Statistical Analysis*

Descriptive statistics were used to summarize patient characteristics and ENE rates. The Cochran-Armitage test for trend was used to evaluate the 5-year trend of cENE and pENE rates for oral cavity cancer. Chi-square tests were used to compare ENE rates between hospital levels and across different cancer sites. Pairwise comparisons of pENE rates across the four HNSCC sites were performed using Chi-square tests with statistical significance set at $p < 0.05$. All statistical analyses were performed using R software (version 4.2.1). A p-value of <0.05 was considered statistically significant.

2.4. *Limitations of Hospital-Level Comparison*

For the hospital-level comparison (medical centers vs. non-medical centers), we acknowledge that these groups may differ in case mix, tumor stage distribution, and referral patterns. Medical centers, as tertiary care institutions, often receive referrals of more advanced or complex cases, which could confound the observed differences in diagnostic gap. Ideally, stage-adjusted or subsite-specific sensitivity analyses would be performed to account for these differences. However, the TCR long-form data structure does not provide sufficient granularity for such stratified analyses at the hospital level. Specifically, the registry does not include detailed T-stage, N-stage, or anatomical subsite information cross-tabulated with hospital-level data in a format that would allow for robust adjusted analyses. Therefore, our hospital-level findings should be interpreted as hypothesis-generating, and residual confounding by case complexity cannot be entirely ruled out. Future studies with more detailed patient-level data would be needed to confirm whether the Quality-Gap Paradox persists after adjustment for stage and other clinical factors.

2.5. *Declaration of AI Tool Usage*

AI-assisted technologies were used strictly for editorial purposes during the manuscript preparation. The WPS Office AI tool was utilized to improve English writing fluency, and the Perplexity platform assisted in checking citation accuracy. The authors reviewed all AI-suggested changes and maintain full responsibility for the integrity and originality of the work.

https://doi.org/10.3390/jpm1602(

3. Results

3.1. Patient Characteristics

A total of 29,830 patients with newly diagnosed HNSCC from 2018 to 2022 were included in the analysis. Oral cavity cancer was the most common site ($n = 27,815$), followed by oropharynx, hypopharynx, and larynx. The majority of patients were male, with a median age in the late 50s.

3.2. Diagnostic Gap Analysis

Across all sites, a significant and persistent diagnostic gap was observed. For oral cavity cancer, the 5-year average cENE rate was 3.8%, while the pENE rate was 13.7%, resulting in an average diagnostic gap of 9.9%. The trend of cENE and pENE rates over the five years is illustrated in Figure 1. The Cochran-Armitage test for trend showed no significant change in the diagnostic gap over the 5-year period ($p = 0.9788$), indicating that the gap did not narrow despite increased awareness following the AJCC eighth edition implementation.

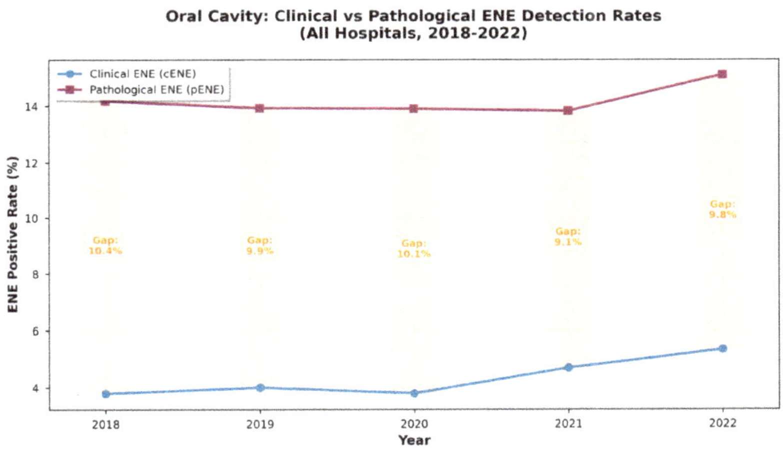

Figure 1. Five-year trend of clinical extranodal extension (cENE) and pathological extranodal extension (pENE) rates in oral cavity cancer patients in Taiwan (2018–2022). The diagnostic gap (pENE rate − cENE rate) remained stable over the study period (Cochran-Armitage trend test, $p = 0.9788$).

3.3. Comparison Across Cancer Sites

A comparison of the 5-year average diagnostic gap across the four major HNSCC sites is shown in Figure 2. Laryngeal cancer exhibited the largest gap (20.8%), followed by hypopharyngeal cancer (20.4%), oropharyngeal cancer (11.5%), and oral cavity cancer (9.9%). Chi-square tests revealed that these differences in pENE rates were statistically significant for most pairwise comparisons (all $p < 0.001$), with the exception of oropharynx versus larynx ($p = 0.74$). Notably, both laryngeal and hypopharyngeal cancers demonstrated gaps approximately twice as large as oral cavity cancer, suggesting site-specific factors influence the diagnostic accuracy of ENE detection.

https://doi.org/10.3390/jpm16020123

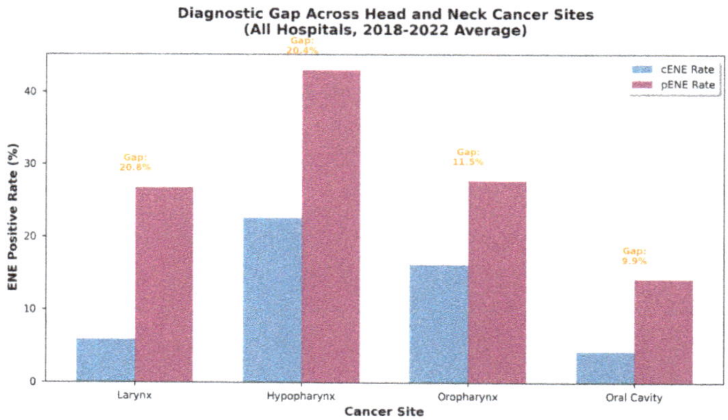

Figure 2. Comparison of the 5-year average diagnostic gap across four major head and neck cancer sites. Laryngeal and hypopharyngeal cancers demonstrated the largest gaps, followed by oropharyngeal and oral cavity cancers.

3.4. *The Quality-Gap Paradox*

When stratified by hospital level, a paradoxical finding emerged. For oral cavity cancer, medical centers had a significantly larger 5-year average diagnostic gap (10.5%) compared to non-medical centers (8.4%). This difference was primarily driven by a higher pENE detection rate in medical centers (14.7% vs. 13.0%), while cENE rates were similar (4.2% vs. 4.6%). Chi-square analysis confirmed that the difference in pENE rates between medical centers and non-medical centers was statistically significant ($\chi^2 = 8.73$, $p = 0.003$), indicating that the observed paradox is not due to chance. This paradox is visualized in Figure 3, which compares the diagnostic gap between the two hospital levels.

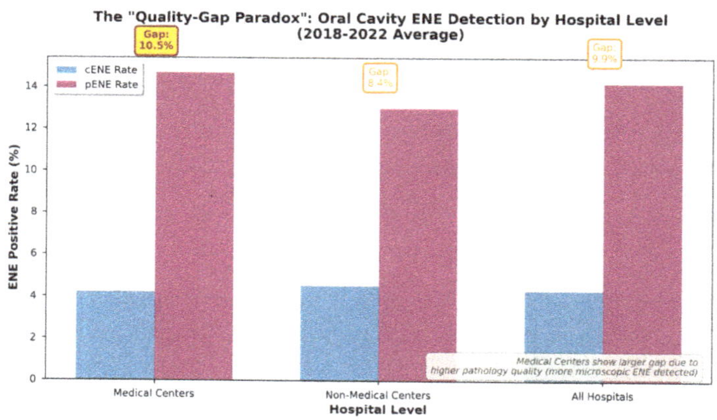

Figure 3. The "Quality-Gap Paradox" in oral cavity cancer. The 5-year average diagnostic gap was significantly larger in medical centers compared to non-medical centers, reflecting higher pathological detection rates.

4. Discussion

This is the first nationwide study in Taiwan to comprehensively evaluate the diagnostic gap between clinical and pathological extranodal extension (ENE) across four major head and neck cancer sites since the implementation of the American Joint Committee on Cancer (AJCC) eighth edition staging system. Our analysis of over 29,000 HNSCC cases from 2018 to 2022 reveals three principal findings with profound implications for personalized

https://doi.org/10.3390/jpm1602C

medicine. First, a significant and persistent diagnostic gap of approximately 10–20% exists, indicating a substantial rate of underdiagnosis of ENE by preoperative imaging. Second, this gap did not narrow over the five-year study period, suggesting that the introduction of ENE as a formal staging criterion has not, by itself, improved the clinical detection rate. Third, and most intriguingly, we identified a "Quality-Gap Paradox," wherein medical centers, despite presumably having more advanced imaging and expertise, exhibited a larger diagnostic gap than non-medical centers. This suggests the gap is driven more by the quality of pathological examination than by deficiencies in clinical assessment. These findings challenge the current "one-size-fits-all" staging paradigm and underscore the urgent need for personalized, risk-adapted treatment strategies in HNSCC.

4.1. The Unwavering Diagnostic Gap: A Barrier to Personalized Risk Stratification

The persistence of the diagnostic gap is a stark reminder of the inherent limitations of current standard-of-care imaging modalities. Our finding of a ~10% gap in oral cavity cancer aligns with a growing body of literature documenting the challenge of accurately detecting ENE preoperatively [5,6]. The core of the issue lies in the distinction between macroscopic ENE, which is often visible on imaging, and microscopic ENE (mENE), where tumor cells breach the lymph node capsule on a microscopic level without causing significant morphological changes [9]. Current imaging techniques are simply not equipped to resolve these microscopic invasions.

From a personalized medicine perspective, this diagnostic gap represents a critical failure in patient stratification. It challenges the current "one-size-fits-all" staging paradigm, where all patients within a given AJCC stage are often considered for similar treatment pathways, despite underlying biological heterogeneity. The inability to preoperatively identify the 10–20% of patients with occult ENE has direct consequences for treatment personalization. The presence of pENE is a major indication for adjuvant therapy intensification. A patient correctly identified with ENE preoperatively might be considered for neoadjuvant systemic therapy, whereas a patient only found to have pENE postoperatively is typically recommended for adjuvant chemoradiation rather than radiation alone. This failure to identify high-risk patients upfront prevents the delivery of truly personalized, risk-adapted care from the outset and subjects patients to a treatment plan based on an incomplete assessment of their disease.

In 2024, the Head and Neck Cancer International Group (HNCIG) published consensus guidelines to standardize the radiological diagnosis of ENE (rENE) [10]. However, these criteria are still based on morphological changes often absent in mENE. Our data, showing no improvement in the gap from 2018 to 2022, suggests that even with heightened awareness, clinicians are hitting a ceiling in diagnostic capability with the tools at hand. This underscores the urgent need for novel technologies that can non-invasively detect microscopic disease, moving beyond anatomical imaging to functional or molecular characterization—a cornerstone of modern personalized oncology.

The lack of improvement in the diagnostic gap over the 5-year study period ($p = 0.9788$ for oral cavity cancer) is particularly noteworthy and warrants careful interpretation. Several factors may explain this stagnation. First, while the AJCC eighth edition heightened awareness of ENE as a critical staging parameter, the fundamental imaging technology (CT and MRI) has not undergone revolutionary advances in spatial resolution during this period. The physical limitations of current imaging modalities in detecting microscopic disease remain unchanged. Second, international standardized criteria for radiological ENE diagnosis were only published in 2024 [10], after our study period, suggesting that earlier years may have suffered from inconsistent interpretation and a lack of consensus on diagnostic thresholds. Third, it is plausible that pathological detection has also improved in

https://doi.org/10.3390/jpm16020123

parallel with clinical awareness, as pathologists became more vigilant in examining lymph nodes for ENE following the AJCC eighth edition's emphasis on this feature. If both clinical and pathological detection improved proportionally, the gap would remain constant even as absolute detection rates increased.

The variation in diagnostic gap across different HNSCC sites is also highly informative and reflects the complex interplay of anatomical, biological, and technical factors. Laryngeal (20.8%) and hypopharyngeal (20.4%) cancers exhibited gaps approximately twice as large as oral cavity cancer (9.9%), and these differences were statistically significant ($p < 0.001$). This disparity likely reflects anatomical and technical factors. Oral cavity tumors are more accessible to direct clinical examination and high-resolution imaging, whereas laryngeal and hypopharyngeal lesions are located in deeper, more complex anatomical regions where lymph nodes may be obscured by surrounding structures, cartilage, and air-tissue interfaces, reducing imaging sensitivity. Furthermore, the lymphatic drainage patterns differ, with laryngeal and hypopharyngeal cancers more frequently involving deep cervical nodes that are challenging to assess radiologically. Interestingly, oropharyngeal and laryngeal cancers had similar gaps ($p = 0.74$), despite differences in anatomical location, suggesting that other factors such as tumor biology or nodal involvement patterns may also play a role.

4.2. The Quality-Gap Paradox: A Multifactorial Hypothesis

Perhaps the most significant finding of our study is the "Quality-Gap Paradox." The observation that medical centers have a consistently larger diagnostic gap in oral cavity cancer (10.46% vs. 8.42%) is statistically significant ($\chi^2 = 8.73$, $p = 0.003$) and, on the surface, counterintuitive. While one might expect superior imaging at these centers to yield a smaller gap, the opposite finding suggests a complex interplay of factors. We propose this paradox is not attributable to a single cause but is likely a multifactorial phenomenon driven by differences in pathological, surgical, and radiological practices.

One primary hypothesis remains the role of pathological scrutiny. Medical centers are more likely to have dedicated head and neck subspecialty pathologists who may perform more meticulous lymph node examination, thereby identifying a higher rate of true pENE, particularly microscopic ENE (mENE), which was missed on imaging [9]. From this perspective, a larger gap could reflect a more thorough and accurate pathological workup, which is crucial for guiding appropriate adjuvant therapy. However, as noted by experts, pathologist skill is not exclusively confined to large centers, and expert practitioners may exist in any setting. Therefore, other factors must be considered.

Alternative or contributing factors may include surgical and radiological procedures. For instance, surgeons at high-volume medical centers might perform more extensive or comprehensive neck dissections, retrieving a higher number of lymph nodes for examination and thus increasing the probability of detecting occult pENE. Furthermore, while medical centers may have advanced imaging technology, the radiological diagnostic criteria for ENE were not internationally standardized until recently [10], potentially leading to variations in interpretation that are independent of hospital level. The observed gap may therefore reflect a combination of more comprehensive surgery and more detailed pathological analysis in medical centers, rather than a simple deficiency in any single area. This reframes the diagnostic gap as an indicator of system-level differences in the cancer care pathway, highlighting the need for further research to dissect the relative contributions of each component. Ultimately, this discussion should not be interpreted as a critique of non-medical centers, but rather as a hypothesis-generating observation that the drivers of staging discordance are complex and multifactorial. The study by Hondorp et al. on clinical-pathologic stage discordance similarly found only moderate agreement, emphasizing that the final pathologic stage remains the gold standard for a reason [11]. Our

https://doi.org/10.3390/jpm1602C

paradox provides a real-world, population-level validation of this principle and suggests that "personalized pathology," characterized by expert, meticulous examination, is as important as personalized imaging or therapy.

An important caveat to our hospital-level analysis is the potential for residual confounding. Medical centers, as tertiary referral institutions, may treat a higher proportion of advanced-stage or complex cases compared to non-medical centers. If medical centers see more patients with advanced nodal disease, this could contribute to a higher pENE detection rate independent of pathological scrutiny. We were unable to perform stage-adjusted analyses due to limitations in the granularity of the TCR data at the hospital level. Therefore, while our findings are suggestive and hypothesis-generating, definitive conclusions about the drivers of the Quality-Gap Paradox will require future studies with patient-level data that allow for adjustment of tumor stage, nodal burden, and other clinical factors.

4.3. Future Directions: The Potential of AI in Bridging the Gap

Our findings highlight the urgent clinical need for advanced tools to bridge the diagnostic gap and improve patient stratification. The diagnostic impasse revealed by our study sets the stage for integrating artificial intelligence (AI) as a potential future solution. The limitations of human interpretation of complex imaging data are precisely the kind of problem that deep learning is poised to solve. Recent landmark studies have shown that AI models can not only predict ENE from CT scans but also quantify the burden of AI-predicted ENE, offering a powerful new prognostic tool [12,13]. This technology holds the promise of moving from a binary clinical assessment to a continuous, quantitative risk score, allowing for truly personalized treatment planning before the first incision is made. While our study did not involve AI analysis, it underscores the necessity of exploring and validating these technologies in future research.

4.4. Clinical Implications and the Path to Implementation

The clinical implications of our findings are immediate and actionable. First, clinicians must maintain a high index of suspicion for occult ENE, even when imaging is negative, particularly in high-risk scenarios (e.g., multiple involved nodes, large nodal size). Second, the "Quality-Gap Paradox" strongly advocates for the centralization of head and neck cancer care, particularly pathology services, to ensure all patients benefit from expert, high-quality diagnosis. Third, our study provides a clear mandate for the clinical validation and adoption of AI-based tools. Healthcare systems and professional societies should invest in the infrastructure and training needed to integrate these technologies into routine clinical workflows.

4.5. Strengths and Limitations

The primary strength of our study is its large, population-based design, which provides a real-world snapshot of the diagnostic gap across an entire country. However, some limitations must be acknowledged. First, the TCR database lacks detailed data on specific imaging protocols or radiologist experience, which could influence cENE detection. Second, we could not correlate findings with patient outcomes, as survival data for this recent cohort is not yet mature. Future studies should link these findings to survival to quantify the prognostic impact of the diagnostic gap. Third, our diagnostic gap metric is a population-level measure and does not assess individual-patient concordance between cENE and pENE. We did not calculate sensitivity, specificity, positive predictive value, or negative predictive value of clinical ENE detection, as this would require patient-level paired data linking each patient's cENE status to their pENE status. The TCR long-form data structure does not provide such paired information at the individual level. Therefore, our findings should be interpreted as reflecting overall under-detection rates rather than

https://doi.org/10.3390/jpm16020123

diagnostic accuracy metrics. Future studies with access to individual patient records could provide complementary insights into the diagnostic performance of imaging at the patient level. Fourth, an inherent limitation of our study design is that pENE data are available only for patients who underwent neck dissection, while cENE data include all patients with imaging assessment. This creates a selection bias, as patients undergoing neck dissection are typically those with clinically or radiologically suspected nodal disease, representing a higher-risk subset of the overall HNSCC population. Consequently, the observed pENE rates may be higher than they would be if all patients underwent surgical pathological examination, and the diagnostic gap may be artificially widened. However, this limitation is unavoidable in real-world registry data, as early-stage patients without clinical nodal involvement do not undergo neck dissection as part of standard care. Despite this, our findings remain clinically meaningful because they reflect the actual diagnostic challenge faced by clinicians: among patients who do undergo surgery and for whom accurate preoperative staging is most critical, imaging still systematically under-detects ENE.

5. Conclusions

In conclusion, our nationwide study reveals a significant and persistent diagnostic gap between cENE and pENE in Taiwan following the implementation of the AJCC eighth edition. This gap, which did not narrow over a five-year period, underscores the inherent limitations of current imaging modalities in detecting microscopic ENE. The existence of a "Quality-Gap Paradox," where medical centers exhibit a larger gap, highlights the crucial role of high-quality pathological examination in accurate staging. These findings challenge the current staging paradigm and signal an urgent need to move from population-based staging to individualized risk assessment. The integration of AI-powered predictive tools, alongside traditional clinical and pathological evaluation, represents the future of personalized HNSCC management, promising to bridge the diagnostic gap and tailor treatment strategies to each patient's unique disease biology.

Author Contributions: Conceptualization, S.-H.H.; methodology, S.-H.H. and H.-F.L.; software, H.-F.L.; validation, S.-H.H.; formal analysis, H.-F.L.; investigation, H.-F.L.; resources, S.-H.H.; data curation, H.-F.L.; writing—original draft preparation, H.-F.L.; writing—review and editing, S.-H.H.; visualization, H.-F.L.; supervision, S.-H.H.; project administration, S.-H.H. All authors have read and agreed to the published version of the manuscript.

Funding: This research received no external funding.

Institutional Review Board Statement: This study utilized data from the Taiwan Cancer Registry, which is a publicly available database containing anonymized and aggregated information. Therefore, no formal ethics review was required. However, the experimental design and study protocol were reviewed and approved by the Institutional Review Board of Mennonite Christian Hospital on 22 January 2026 (IRB No. 26-01-007), confirming that the study complies with relevant institutional and national guidelines.

Informed Consent Statement: Patient consent was waived as this study analyzed publicly available, de-identified, and aggregated statistical data from the Taiwan Cancer Registry. The data cannot be linked to individual patients.

Data Availability Statement: The data presented in this study are available on request from the Taiwan Cancer Registry. Restrictions apply to the availability of these data, which were used under license for the current study, and so are not publicly available. The aggregated data analyzed are presented within the manuscript.

Conflicts of Interest: The authors declare no conflicts of interest.

https://doi.org/10.3390/jpm16020

erences

Bernier, J.; Cooper, J.S.; Pajak, T.F.; van Glabbeke, M.; Bourhis, J.; Forastiere, A.; Ozsahin, E.M.; Jacobs, J.R.; Jassem, J.; Ang, K.K.; et al. Defining risk levels in locally advanced head and neck cancers: A comparative analysis of concurrent postoperative radiation plus chemotherapy trials of the EORTC (#22931) and RTOG (#9501). *Head Neck* **2005**, *27*, 843–850. [CrossRef] [PubMed]
Huang, S.H.; Chernock, R.; O"Sullivan, B.; Fakhry, C. Assessment criteria and clinical implications of extranodal extension in head and neck cancer. In Proceedings of the American Society of Clinical Oncology Educational Book, Virtual, 4–8 June 2021; Volume 41, pp. 265–278.
Mermod, M.; Tolstonog, G.; Simon, C.; Monnier, Y. Extracapsular spread in head and neck squamous cell carcinoma: A systematic review and meta-analysis. *Oral Oncol.* **2016**, *62*, 60–71. [CrossRef] [PubMed]
Amin, M.B.; Greene, F.L.; Edge, S.B.; Compton, C.C.; Gershenwald, J.E.; Brookland, R.K.; Meyer, L.; Gress, D.M.; Byrd, D.R.; Winchester, D.P. The Eighth Edition AJCC Cancer Staging Manual: Continuing to build a bridge from a population-based to a more "personalized" approach to cancer staging. *CA Cancer J. Clin.* **2017**, *67*, 93–99. [CrossRef] [PubMed]
Park, S.I.; Guenette, J.P.; Suh, C.H.; Hanna, G.J.; Chung, S.R.; Baek, J.H.; Lee, J.H.; Choi, Y.J. The diagnostic performance of CT and MRI for detecting extranodal extension in patients with head and neck squamous cell carcinoma: A systematic review and diagnostic meta-analysis. *Eur. Radiol.* **2021**, *31*, 2048–2061. [CrossRef] [PubMed]
Abdel-Halim, C.N.; Rosenberg, T.; Dyrvig, A.-K.; Høilund-Carlsen, P.F.; Sørensen, J.A.; Rohde, M.; Godballe, C. Diagnostic accuracy of imaging modalities in detection of histopathological extranodal extension: A systematic review and meta-analysis. *Oral Oncol.* **2021**, *114*, 105169. [CrossRef] [PubMed]
Chou, C.-W.; Lin, C.-R.; Chung, Y.-T.; Tang, C.-S. Epidemiology of oral cancer in Taiwan: A population-based cancer registry study. *Cancers* **2023**, *15*, 2175. [CrossRef] [PubMed]
Rumgay, H.; Nethan, S.T.; Shah, R.; Vignat, J.; Ayo-Yusuf, O.; Chaturvedi, P.; Guerra, E.N.S.; Gupta, P.C.; Gupta, R.; Liu, S.; et al. Global burden of oral cancer in 2022 attributable to smokeless tobacco and areca nut consumption: A population attributable fraction analysis. *Lancet Oncol.* **2024**, *25*, 1413–1423. [CrossRef] [PubMed]
Chohan, S.; Zaheer, S. Pathological extranodal extension in head and neck cancer: A prognostic biomarker with therapeutic ramifications and diagnostic pitfalls. *Pathol. Res. Pract.* **2025**, *256*, 156183. [CrossRef] [PubMed]
Henson, C.; Abou-Foul, A.K.; Yu, E.; Glastonbury, C.; Huang, S.H.; King, A.D.; Lydiatt, W.M.; McDowell, L.; Nagelschneider, A.A.; Nankivell, P.C.; et al. Criteria for the diagnosis of extranodal extension detected on radiological imaging in head and neck cancer: Head and Neck Cancer International Group consensus recommendations. *Lancet Oncol.* **2024**, *25*, e297–e307. [CrossRef] [PubMed]
Hondorp, B.; Punjabi, N.; Macias, D.; Liu, Y.; Frank, E.; Kim, P.D.; Inman, J.C. Patterns of Discordance Between Clinical and Pathologic Stage in Head and Neck Cancer. *Laryngoscope* **2024**, *134*, 4284–4291. [CrossRef] [PubMed]
Ye, Z.; Mojahed-Yazdi, R.; Zapaishchykova, A.; Tak, D.; Mahootiha, M.; Pardo, J.C.C.; Zielke, J.; Zha, Y.; Guthier, C.; Tishler, R.B.; et al. Automated lymph node and extranodal extension assessment improves risk stratification in oropharyngeal carcinoma. *J. Clin. Oncol.* **2026**, *44*, 386–399. [CrossRef] [PubMed]
Kann, B.H.; Likitlersuang, J.; Bontempi, D.; Ye, Z.; Aneja, S.; Bakst, R.; Kelly, H.R.; Juliano, A.F.; Payabvash, S.; Guenette, J.P.; et al. Screening for extranodal extension in HPV-associated oropharyngeal carcinoma: Evaluation of a CT-based deep learning algorithm in patient data from a multicentre, randomised de-escalation trial. *Lancet Digit. Health* **2023**, *5*, e360–e369. [CrossRef] [PubMed] [PubMed Central]

https://doi.org/10.3390/jpm16020123

MDPI AG
Grosspeteranlage 5
4052 Basel
Switzerland
Tel.: +41 61 683 77 34

Journal of Personalized Medicine Editorial Office
E-mail: jpm@mdpi.com
www.mdpi.com/journal/jpm

www.ingramcontent.com/pod-product-compliance
Lightning Source LLC
Chambersburg PA
CBHW041954260926
51850CB00019B/2732

9783725880331